MASTERING RESISTANCE

THE GUILFORD FAMILY THERAPY SERIES
ALAN S. GURMAN, EDITOR

MASTERING RESISTANCE

A practical guide to family therapy

Carol M. Anderson and Susan Stewart

University of Pittsburgh
Western Psychiatric Institute and Clinic

Foreword by Lyman C. Wynne

THE GUILFORD PRESS
New York   London

© 1983 The Guilford Press
A Division of Guilford Publications, Inc.
200 Park Avenue South, New York, N.Y. 10003

Printed in the United States of America

LIBRARY OF CONGRESS CATALOGING IN PUBLICATION DATA
Anderson, Carol M., 1939–
  Mastering resistance.

  (The Guilford family therapy series)
  Bibliography: p.
  Includes index.
  1. Family psychotherapy. 2. Resistance (Psychoanaly-
sis) I. Stewart, Susan, 1940–   II. Title.
III. Series.
RC488.5.A475   1983   616.89'156   82-21033
ISBN 0-89862-044-9

Foreword

This book will have a wide appeal for family therapists and theorists. First and foremost, the practicing clinician in family and marital therapy will find it the first volume that focuses exclusively but fully on the difficulties and impasses of therapy. Other books have expounded on many facets of a particular school of therapy, and still others have discussed treatment of certain classes of family problems. Nowhere, until now, has there been a thorough stocktaking of the kinds of stalling, digressions, evasions—the resistances that actually confront family therapists, and to which they contribute, from the first phone call to the termination of treatment. This diversity of problems encompasses all components of the therapeutic system —the family, the therapist, and the institutional context. Some of the topics have been quite neglected in previous writings on family therapy, particularly resistances in the form of challenges to the therapist's competence, and the resistances produced by helping systems—therapists, agencies, and institutions. For each sharply specified treatment problem, a series of suggestions are offered, drawing upon essentially all prevailing schools of family therapy, with numerous examples indicating when each suggestion may be relevant. This aspect of the volume will be especially helpful to therapists who are just entering this field and who are befuddled by the diversity of approaches proposed by different authors. Here, each school is put in its place, so to speak—each having its place, but none alone providing the repertory of skills that may be needed.

Teachers and supervisors of family therapy will find this volume a valuable resource unless they are dedicated to only one school of therapy. Even for experienced therapists who have some familiarity with the total field, the authors provide sensible suggestions that are simply omitted from standard textbooks. For example, the discussion of how to deal with resistances to the formation of contracts with families includes many points that will be useful for most supervisors.

No doubt family theoreticians will be the ones most likely to contest the concepts formulated by the authors. In some quarters, the concept of resistance is clearly resisted, but, I believe, as the result of misunderstanding. Anderson and Stewart begin with a splendid review of the literature on the topic, not only in the field of family therapy but also in the literature of other types of therapy in which the concept has been used. Perhaps the most common reason given for avoiding the term "resistance" is that it is often mistakenly understood to be a function only of the client or family. Instead, it is argued, the inept therapist should correct his/her technique. Anderson and Stewart point out that resistance can be identified in any component of the therapeutic system; above all, the interaction and fine tuning of the three spheres of family, therapist, and context become the task in mastering resistance. Another common notion about resistance is that it is a way for the therapist to rationalize therapeutic failure. This pragmatic volume good-humoredly recognizes failures, but rationalization is conspicuous by its absence. Still another viewpoint is that everything ultimately fits together so that resistance really cannot exist. The latter is strictly a philosophical point of view that has little relevance for the practicing clinician who is stuck in a therapeutic impasse.

I believe that the authors cogently establish the point that these various objections to the concept of resistance stem substantially from a failure to use the term systemically. That is, resistance is any property of the *therapeutic system,* including the family members, the therapist, and the context in which therapy takes place, that inteferes with achieving the family's goals for therapy. From this standpoint, resistance, as the authors suggest, "is alive and well and living under an assumed name." One could add that resistance is a thorn that by any other name pricks as deep. Additionally, as a universal and necessary component of change, in therapy and otherwise, resistance emerges from this volume with functions both positive and distressing.

Lyman C. Wynne

Preface

Family therapy is one of the most powerful and exciting approaches to psychotherapy. It offers a new way of understanding behavior and the opportunity to change patterns of interaction which have persisted for years, if not generations. It also presents a real challenge to those who would become and remain competent and creative practitioners. While family therapy theories are not difficult to grasp, the practice of family therapy is complex. In fact, when one of the authors complained of difficulty persuading residents to take family cases, a recent graduate of the residency program told her flatly, "Residents don't do family therapy because it's too hard!"

As teachers of family therapy, watching year after year as students struggle to put theories into practice, we have sometimes been inclined to agree that family therapy is too complex for beginners. They lose an inordinate number of cases before, during, and after the first interview; they encounter an unusual number of families who question their credentials and attack their competence; they become bogged down in hopeless impasses as family members fail to change and/or continue to point blaming fingers at one another. In short, they run headlong into *resistance*. Those new to family therapy are not the only ones who experience problems with resistance. Experienced family therapists also find themselves complaining from time to time about resistant families who don't want treatment, don't want to change, and, worst of all, are hostile toward their therapists in the process.

Resistance is a major component of any form of psychotherapy. In family therapy, however, dealing effectively with resistance is complicated by a number of factors: the number of people involved in the therapy; the variety of subtle forms in which resistance appears in family systems; and the ease with which therapists can find themselves perpetuating or even encouraging a family's tendencies to resist change. While resistance is natural and inevitable, beginning family therapists tend to be surprised and put off when it occurs. They feel hurt by challenges to their competence and too easily accept a family's refusal to cooperate at face value. Even experienced family therapists, while hardly surprised by resistance, have problems coping with it effectively. They become discouraged by the prevalence and persistence of resistant behaviors. When resistance is high or the therapists' energy is low, they become caught in creative backwaters, unable to develop a helpful perspective for a difficult case, or a novel technique to unbalance the status quo. All things considered, learning to recognize, understand, and cope with the complex ways in which families express resistance is often the most difficult task in becoming and/or remaining an effective family therapist.

In the "forewarned is forearmed" tradition, the purpose of this book is to help family therapists to anticipate common expressions of resistance, and to be prepared with alternative strategies for coping with them. It is intended as a cookbook on resistance in family therapy which we hope will both short-circuit the long and trying process of putting theory and practice together and offer relief to any therapist frustrated by a difficult therapeutic situation. It can be used by beginning family therapists to obtain ideas for specific interventions until they have developed their own repetoire of interventions, or by experienced family therapists suffering from "therapist fatigue" until they can rediscover their own energy and creativity. In either case, the book is intended for use primarily by students and practitioners who do not have access to those treatment and training centers in which the major approaches to family therapy have been or are being developed. Such centers provide direction and leadership for the field, but are usually quite different from the circumstances under which most family therapists practice. Those practicing in less ideal surroundings often need help that is not available in the form of a resident guru or a team behind the mirror.

The concepts and interventions in this book are derived from the clinical experience of the authors, their colleagues, and their students. All clinical examples are based on actual cases, although names and identifying data of families, and sometimes even therapists, have been changed to protect the innocent and, on occasion, the guilty. The authors have attempted to avoid taking any particular theoretical approach, preferring to reflect the eclectic and often pragmatic way in which family therapy is practiced.

Chapter 1 traces the development of the concept of resistance and provides a brief overview of the ways in which resistance is now viewed in the field. A broad definition of resistance is offered, one that includes all behaviors of the family, the therapist, and the therapeutic system that operate to inhibit the family from becoming involved in therapy, or, once the family is engaged, that prevent or delay change. Chapter 2 deals with initial resistances, those that occur in the beginning stage of treatment when families are not sure they want to come to therapy at all, much less change. Chapter 3 considers resistances to the treatment contract, that is, challenges to the boundaries of treatment. Chapter 4 deals with challenges to the therapist's professional or personal credentials, those direct or indirect questions about the therapist's marital status or training that feel like frontal assaults to new therapists. Chapter 5 is concerned with the resistances that come up after therapist and family have settled into ongoing treatment. It includes those resistances common to all treatment (intellectualization, denial) and those that are more particular to family therapy (collusions, secrets, and pseudohostility). Finally, Chapter 6 examines the resistances created or sustained by therapists and by the systems within which therapists operate.

A word of caution is in order here. This book offers a range of survival strategies for therapists to use in situations that could otherwise cause them anxiety, frustration, or resentment. The key to successful application of any of the strategies is an accurate assessment by the therapist of the nature and function of the resistance in any given situation. No matter how clever a strategy may be, it won't work unless the therapist has chosen it appropriately. Applying an intervention inappropriately is like the March Hare who, having tried to fix the Mad Hatter's watch with butter, stated regretfully when it didn't work, "It was the best butter, too, the very best butter!"

The forms in which families can offer their therapists both resistance and the opportunity to create change are virtually infinite. As the reader will note, this book contains suggestions for avoiding resistance, meeting it head on, or even using it as a vehicle for change. Although the suggestions are many and varied, they are only a fraction of the options that become available once therapists are comfortable enough to be able to think on their feet. Nevertheless, coping creatively with resistance, whether by using the strategies suggested in this book or by devising one's own, will always require that the family therapist continuously exercise those qualities described by Douglas Hofstadter as the abilities of intelligence:

to respond to situations very flexibly;
to take advantage of fortuitous circumstances;
to make sense out of ambiguous or contradictory messages;
to recognize the relative importance of different elements of a situation;
to find similarities between situations despite differences which may separate them;
to draw distinctions between situations despite similarities which may link them;
to synthesize new concepts by taking old concepts and putting them together in new ways;
to come up with ideas which are novel. (1979, p. 26)

The authors wish to acknowledge the contributions of the staff and students of the Family Therapy Clinic in the Department of Psychiatry, University of Pittsburgh, along with the contributions of other members of the faculty, Peter B. Henderson, MD, Paul Appelbaum, MD, Michel

Hersen, PhD, Paulina McCullough, MSW, and Paul Pilkonis, PhD. In addition, the authors wish to thank the Chairman of the Department, Thomas Detre, MD, for his support of this project. Contributions were also made by the students in the Certificate Program in Family Therapy of the Smith College School for Social Work, and its Director, Gerry Schamess. Valuable comments and criticisms of early drafts were made by Michael Goldstein, Alan Gurman, Jerrold Maxmen, Monica McGoldrick, and Froma Walsh. Finally, special thanks go to Selma Stone who typed the manuscript, and Joanne Cobb who ran the office while Mrs. Stone was otherwise employed.

Contents

1. Resistance

Taking a new step, uttering a new word, is what people
fear most.—Fëdor Dostoevski

Introduction

Resistance to change in general and resistance to being influenced in particular always occurs when individuals, groups, and systems are required by circumstances to alter their established behaviors. Unless people are immediately persuaded by overwhelming evidence that a change in their behavior is necessary or beneficial, such as responding to a fire by exiting from a building, they will resist change in the status quo. Business executives seeking to introduce new marketing techniques, doctors seeking to heal their patients, parents seeking to teach their children manners, all who seek to bring about change experience resistance to their efforts.

Being in the business of bringing about change, psychotherapists encounter resistance continuously. However great the distress people feel, they resist asking for help, and having asked for help, they resist being influenced by the professionals they have employed to help them. This resistance may be expressed overtly, through missed appointments or blatant refusals to comply with the terms of the therapeutic contract; but more frequently it is expressed covertly through a failure to share relevant information, an apparent inability to understand the therapist's comments, or pervasive and persistent refusals to give up old expectations or behaviors.

On the surface, resistance in psychotherapy would appear to be an irrational process which serves no useful purpose. What possible reason could there be for people to request help and then behave in ways that sabotage the helping process? It would seem logical that individuals in pain would be only too happy to do anything necessary to alleviate the distress which drove them to seek therapy in the first place. Yet, irrational as it may seem, resistance is universal.

Because it is so universal, therapists, regardless of their theoretical orientation or the therapeutic modality they practice, must learn to expect and deal with resistance or their efforts to bring about change will be defeated. Mastering resistance, however, is not a simple task. Most therapists have chosen their profession because they are invested in helping

1

people. In return for their concern and good will, therapists hope for and expect gratitude, or at least respect. Sometimes gratitude and respect are forthcoming; but when the efforts of therapists to help are met with apparent indifference, skepticism, or even outright hostility, their reactions are not always rational ones. Resistance *feels* personal to therapists. However well they know that resistance is to be expected, when they encounter it, therapists can become frustrated, insecure, or even actively rejecting of their patients. In turn, they unwittingly communicate their anger or frustration to resistant patients, fostering further resistance and perpetuating a negative spiral of interactions likely to end in treatment failures. Young or inexperienced therapists are particularly vulnerable to personalizing resistance, interpreting it as rejection or as confirmation of their lack of skill. These therapists, therefore, are the most likely to become flustered, hostile, or hopeless when they encounter it. Even experienced therapists can be vulnerable to or trapped by the negative effects of resistance. While they may be somewhat less likely to take it personally, they often find that the cumulative impact of coping with ongoing resistance can result in a loss of creative energy and an increase in therapist fatigue. These factors can result in the same tendencies to give up or retaliate that are common to beginners.

While all therapists encounter resistance, the resistance experienced by family therapists is particularly challenging. Since most families present with one symptomatic member, other family members may fail to see the relevance of involving the whole family, or fear that requests for such family involvement amount to the therapist's blaming them for their problem member's difficulties. Dealing effectively with the resistance stimulated by these perceptions is complicated by the fact that some family members are likely to be more invested in change than others, that some members will resist overtly and others covertly, and that the overt resistance of some members may serve a covert function for others.

Throughout the course of treatment, therapists must deal with each member's multiple expressions of resistance to change while simultaneously being alert to the function of resistances for the family as a whole. If therapists are inexperienced, tired, or both, these factors can combine to prevent much from happening. For example, the parents of a 23-year-old man requested treatment, complaining that their oldest son had dropped out of college several years earlier despite excellent grades. He had subsequently lost his job as a laborer, and for the past several years had limited his social contacts to family members and his activities to watching television in the basement. The family appeared eager for help, yet despite specific instructions to bring all five of their children, they arrived at the initial interview with only the identified patient and their youngest child, a 9-year-old daughter, claiming that their older adolescent and young adult children were unavailable. Despite the therapist's pressure and the family's overt promises of compliance, not only did the identified patient's brothers and sisters fail to attend the second session, but the identified patient failed to show up as well. These parents passively accepted their children's expression of ambivalent or negative feelings toward therapy as an absolute refusal to attend, and did nothing to encourage them to do so. While this parental behavior also reflected the larger problem these parents had in taking control of their family, further discussion revealed clues that they, too, had ambivalence about therapy in general, and the attendance of their children in particular. It became clear that their children had been critical about the way in which they were handling the patient and that they feared the confrontations that might occur if the entire family became involved. When the therapist pursued these feelings, the parents failed to see how their own behavior contributed to their children's resistance and how these issues were operating to discourage change. In fact, the father stated, "I don't understand what happens. We talk about what we need to do, but we just can't manage to do it." The frustrated therapist soon gave up her efforts to include the children, fearing that if she pushed these parents too far, their passivity would turn to hostility. While the case was not lost altogether, change was minimal and slow in coming.

In this case, the overt resistance of the children served a covert purpose for their apparently cooperative parents. Such passive resistances are relatively easy to manage once therapists have learned to recognize them. But not all resistances by family members are so lacking in overt hostility. In fact, the resistance of family members is frequently expressed by skeptical or hostile remarks and direct challenges of the therapist's competence. Consider the following example: A few years ago, a successful businessman phoned our family therapy clinic. Revealing nothing about himself or his problem, he demanded to know if the clinician answering his call had read several volumes by prominent authors on the subject of eating disorders. Assured that the clinician had indeed acquainted herself with the literature, he next mentioned several prominent treatment facilities at which he had already had consultations, alluded to a personal relationship with the Chairman of the Department of Psychiatry, the clinician's ultimate superior, and demanded to know the clinician's professional and personal credentials. This man, so accustomed to success in business, was experiencing failure in his efforts to cure his daughter's anorexia nervosa. Bringing in expensive consultants to view the problem and give advice, his successful method of coping professionally, wasn't working. Worse, his last consultant had suggested family therapy, intimating the family might be in some way involved in the problem. His manner was irritable, negative, and challenging. He and his family desperately needed help, yet his behavior seemed calculated to alienate the very people whom he hoped might be able to provide it.

One could scarcely have blamed the therapist who answered this man's call for help if she had been put off, and even if she had found some way of discouraging him from using her services. She *felt* under attack. She felt as though her worth was being questioned, her competence challenged. At such times, it is hard for therapists to see the fear and frustration inherent in behavior of this sort. It is far easier to become angry or hurt, or to respond in kind, or to dismiss the caller as insufficiently motivated to benefit from treatment.

Therapists must learn not to personalize such evasions or attacks. In particular, therapists must understand that resistance in therapy is only rarely related to their qualities as therapists per se, but rather is part of a universal and natural resistance to change and resistance to being influenced which has many positive functions. Without a certain amount of resistance to change, all social systems would dissolve into chaos and confusion, responding helter-skelter to every input received. Without a certain amount of resistance to change, a family would be unable to provide the stability necessary for its members to grow and develop. Without a certain amount of resistance to being influenced, families and individuals would be converted by every medicine man, commercial, or talk show "expert" that happened to bend their collective ear. Resistance, in other words, can be a sign of health and good judgment. As Lynn Hoffman says, resistance might better be called persistence. Whatever it is called, somehow therapists must attend to the process that occurs when they attempt to influence the patients and families that seek their help.

A brief history of resistance and healing

Resistance as a phenomenon accompanying the healing process has a history which appears to extend back to the earliest human cultures. Based on observations of contemporary shamans and priests, it seems that those performing healing roles have long understood that unless they inducted the patient into the healing process, the patient would "resist" getting well. The rituals of indoctrination used by shamans often involve complicated procedures designed to establish an atmosphere of expectancy, that is, to lead the patient to expect to be cured (Frank, 1961). The shamans are apparently astute at assessing who would respond to their methods and knowledgeable about how to use rituals to maximize the power of that response. After they induct the patient into the process, usually by having the patient perform certain ceremonial tasks, they use a ritual to bring about change, such as spitting out a piece of blood-covered material which is then labeled the cause of the patient's distress. Those who expect to be cured frequently are. The shamans clearly achieve healing by manipulating expectations and perceptions.

Relieving physical and mental distress through the manipulation of psychological processes has continued throughout history into the present. Today, in our culture, it is usually called psychotherapy, except when it occurs in fringe religious movements when it is called faith healing. It has acquired some scientific trappings along the way and a lot of speculation about whether, how, and why it works.

Sigmund Freud was one of the first to apply scientific methods to the study of achieving change through the manipulation of psychological processes (Freud, 1900/1952). He rapidly discovered that patients who requested that he relieve their distress resisted revealing their thoughts and feelings, resisted his interpretations, and resisted exploring their relationship to him. Freud believed that resistances, like defense mechanisms, served to protect patients from the intense anxiety inherent in becoming aware of their unresolved intrapsychic conflicts or unacceptable thoughts and impulses. He believed that despite their desire for help, patients were reluctant to give up their symptoms because the symptoms themselves were their method of maintaining an otherwise threatened intrapsychic equilibrium.

Given this concept of resistance, it is easy to see why it became one of the cornerstones of psychoanalytic practice. As one psychoanalyst expressed it to the authors, "Resistance is all." Clearly, in the psychoanalytic approach to treatment, resistance is not something to be overcome to get to the "real" issues of therapy, since working through resistance *is* the therapy. Defined as "all those conscious or unconscious emotions, attitudes, ideas, thoughts or actions which operate against the progress of therapy" (Greenson, 1967, p. 60), resistance is generally regarded as residing in the patient's unconscious and as being expressed in the context of the transference. Analysts believe that in treatment, patients project the unresolved conflicts originally experienced in early relationships onto their relationship with the therapist. As therapy seeks to explore these projections, old conflicts are relived and anxiety increases. Said Frieda Fromm-Reichmann: "The same source which motivated the patient's original dissociative and repressive processes, that is, his anxiety is also the main reason for the resistance" (Fromm-Reichmann, 1950, p. 110). Resistance means the reactivation, outside the patients' awareness, of the motivating powers which were responsible for the mental patients' original pathogenic dissociative and repressive processes (Fromm-Reichmann, 1950). While patients may be conscious of being reluctant to reveal certain thoughts or impulses, they are not aware of the meaning of their resistance until it has been worked through in the therapeutic process.

In psychoanalytic approaches, then, much of the therapy consists of analyzing when, what, why, and how the patient resists exposing his/her thoughts and feelings, and the significance of what such resistances reveal about the patient's problems. In other words, psychoanalysts use an exploration of the patient's natural resistance to achieve understanding and change. Traditionally, change is thought to occur as a result of the insight gained when the patient's resistance is lifted and the patient is freed from his/her pathological conflicts. Currently, however, there are variations within the analytic community on this view of change, and even in the definition of resistance. Some would now say that it is the experience of the therapeutic relationship, rather than insight per se that allows patients to give up their resistance and symptomatology. Further, while resistance was at one time viewed as entirely in the patient, with his/her internal reality being projected onto the transference relationship, currently, some psychoanalysts would stress a more interactional view of resistance, including a focus on the potential realistic basis of resistance such as therapist error (Greenson, 1967). Nevertheless, although specific definitions may vary, the process of *working through* resistance remains central to psychoanalytically oriented therapies. For this reason, therapy of this sort is a time-consuming process in which change is only possible when patients are sufficiently motivated to withstand the pain of insight and the slow process of reworking old conflicts in a new relationship.

The psychoanalytic movement is largely responsible for a general acceptance of psychotherapy as a legitimate means of helping people cope more effectively with their lives. However, as has been stated, the process of working through resistance takes a great deal of time and money, and requires that the patient have a serious commitment to the therapeutic process. Because these requirements restrict the appropriateness of therapy to a very select population, the demand arose for therapies which could be applied to a wider range of patients in shorter periods of time for less money. In fact, efforts to develop short-term therapies date back to the time of Freud himself, specifically involving two of his followers, Sandor Ferenczi and Otto Rank. Both recognized that to speed up therapy, the therapist would have to apply different techniques to resistance.

Ferenczi recommended that therapists become more active in forming relationships with their patients. He suggested that therapists facilitate the development of patient trust through hugging, kissing, and nonerotic fondling (Ferenczi, 1950). While he quickly abandoned physical touching of the patient for fear that it was a potentially problematic technique, he did point the way to therapists becoming more active in overcoming patient resistance to change, going so far as to forbid his patients to relieve tension through body movements or masturbation. Otto Rank also attempted to develop ways of facilitating the therapeutic relationship which might in turn minimize resistance. He recommended that the therapist engage the "will" of the patient (Rank, 1947). Presumably, he was implying that resistance would be overcome more quickly if the patient's motivation was exploited and his/her will were engaged in the therapeutic process.

Currently, the response of psychodynamically oriented therapists to the demand for less extended and expensive treatment approaches is a shortened form of treatment variously called short-term dynamic psy-chotherapy or psychoanalytic psychotherapy. These forms of therapy are based on the insights and basic theoretical principles of classic psychoanalysis (Marmor, 1979) but their approach to resistance is quite different. Certainly, working through resistance is no longer viewed as the only or even the most important way of coping with it. For example, two contemporary leaders in the short-term psychodynamic therapy movement, Peter Sifneos (1973) and James Mann (1973), appear to handle resistance first by avoiding the need to deal with it as much as possible, and second by overcoming it with direct and massive confrontation. Both advocate a screening process which would seem to select the healthiest, least resistant patients. Patients selected for this type of therapy are described as "highly motivated, intelligent people with demonstrated ego strengths and interpersonal skills . . . those who can bear the pain (anxiety), without disintegrating or terminating prematurely" (Burke, White, & Havens, 1979, p. 177). Thus, the need to deal with resistance is in part avoided by choosing patients who are less likely to "need" to resist. In fact, one suggested selection criterion is a patient's ability to accept and respond to an interpretation in the first session.

This rigorous selection process also insures that patients will have a greater ability to withstand the therapist's head-on confrontations of what remaining resistances arise. This point is crucial since these therapists directly confront patients with interpretations which include immediate references to their past object relationships, their current relationships, and the transference itself. Discussing Peter Sifneos's technique, Burke and his colleagues (1979) state, "The interpretation is made in such a forceful way that the patient has the choice of either fighting him, acknowledging that it is true, or quitting treatment" (p. 178). While the concept of resistance is not directly addressed in these approaches, the suggested methods of intervention clearly imply it is a factor which must be avoided and/or overcome in order to create rapid change.

Other therapists conducting short-term dynamic psychotherapy are more explicit about the issue of resistance, advocating active and direct confrontation from the very beginning of therapy (Davanloo, 1980; Malan, 1980). Davanloo early and persistently confronts resistances, utilizes the transference and makes connections between the therapeutic relationship and those relationships in the patient's current and past life. Using this technique, he reports symptom relief and basic personality changes in a maximum of 25 sessions, with gains apparently maintained for at least five years (Davanloo, 1980). These results are particularly impressive since Davanloo specifically recommends his technique for patients with severe and long-standing psychoneurotic and characterologic problems. Malan largely attributes these good results to the fact that this technique, while firmly grounded on psychoanalytic principles, does not involve responding to the increasing resistance of the patients with increasing passivity on the part of the therapist (Malan, 1980). Resistance is central and is dealt with relentlessly.

Resistance: Alive and well and living under an assumed name

Psychodynamically oriented short-term therapies can be assumed to have inherited their concept of resistance from the classic analytic tradition, as they have their other underlying principles. Other forms of brief therapy, however, have less clearly defined notions about what resistance is and how it should be handled. Therapeutic techniques and procedures which could serve the purpose of avoiding or minimizing resistance are often described without any specific mention of resistance. In fact, references to resistance are often made obliquely, tacitly acknowledging its existence without attempting to define it.

For instance, surprisingly little has been written about resistance in the behavioral therapy literature, which usually is prolific on almost every subject. Based on social learning theory, this approach regards psychotherapy as primarily an educational, skill-building process (Shelton & Ackerman, 1974). Therapists teach problem solving and interpersonal skills by modeling, shaping, and task assignment. They desensitize patients to anxiety-provoking situations and promote change through the effective use of positive and negative reinforcements, that is, the management of contingencies. Therapeutic strategies are based on the assumption that humans are rational beings who will engage in behaviors only so long as those behaviors are to their advantage. Presumably, people who come to therapy find their behaviors no longer rewarding and thus are ready to change.

When they talk about resistance at all, behavioral therapists tend to talk about it in terms of noncompliance, that is, for some reason the patient fails to carry out the assignment given by the therapist with the result that the anticipated change in his/her behavior fails to occur. Most of the techniques described by behavioral therapists to increase compliance are ones which would serve to avoid the emergence of resistance. It is generally the responsibility of therapists to insure compliance by a number of techniques, such as involving the client and prescribing appropriate tasks (Hersen, 1979). For instance, Martin and Worthington (in press) suggest prescribing effective homework assignments, specifying that tasks be logically related to the goal of therapy, suggestions be presented in a way the client will accept them, tasks be kept small, concrete, specific, and simple, and clients be involved in devising the assignment. In fact, several behavioral authors have stressed this last point, that is, the need to actively involve the client in the process of his/her treatment. In discussing noncompliance with homework, for instance, Shelton and Ackerman (1974) cite the two most common reasons for problems as the lack of explicit instructions and lack of relevance of the task to the client's needs. They state, "The more the client participates in the endeavor, the greater his chances of making desired changes. Ideally, the client and therapist coparticipate in treatment; they work together to clarify, select and attain the goals of therapy" (p. 14).

The stress on involving the client in the treatment process often extends to a specific effort to deemphasize the role of the therapist in causing change, and decreasing the obviousness of the therapist's attempts to influence the client. This emphasis appears to be based on a theme of the social psychological literature that change attributed to self is more likely to be maintained than change attributed to external agents (Kopel & Arkowitz, 1975; Kanfer, 1975; Martin & Worthington, in press). As is noted by Hoyt, Henley, and Collins (1972), "internal attribution, whether correct or incorrect, will maximize the probability that the act will produce lasting personal change" (p. 209). Client involvement can also be used to insure that the task or directive is relevant to his/her needs. Noncompliance is thus avoided by anticipating with patients the problems they will have complying with tasks or directive (Martin & Worthington, in press).

This is not to say that there has been no direct attention to resistance in the behavioral literature. Hersen (1981), for example, acknowledges resistance and complains that it is too often met with oversimplified explanations of operant conditioning, bypassing the need to understand the phenomena or come up with any strategies of overcoming resistance which do not depend on the patient being unambivalent about change. Wilson and Evans (1977) suggest resistance in behavioral therapy can be said to exist when either of two phenomena are encountered: when therapists evoke strong antipathies in clients, or when therapists are unable to elicit particular responses from patients. When the cause of resistance is an unspoken resentment of the therapist, they suggest that assertiveness training is in order to encourage its expression and thus its management. When clients repeatedly fail to follow through on assignments, they suggest a logical analysis of the possible causes. They tend to believe that the required behavior either is not in the client's behavioral repertoire, or evokes more anxiety than can be counteracted by the eliciting power of the therapist. In either case, they suggest a more gradual behavioral shaping process to cope with such resistances. Mahoney (1974) is one of the few behaviorists who specifically deals with resistance to being influenced by the therapist, a resistance which he calls "countercontrol," in which the patient behaves in the opposite direction of the established contingency. He cites, for instance, an example of a 6-year-old boy who wet the bed more when doughnuts were given for dry nights. He maintains that the likelihood of such negative responses to assignments are influenced by the absence of choice, the conspicuousness of the therapist's coercive efforts, and the presence of noncompliant role models.

At least one set of behaviorally oriented authors has attempted to construct a model of resistance which could be researched. Munjack and Oziel (1978) propose five types of resistance, including misunderstanding or skill deficit on the part of the patient; lack of motivation or a low expectation of success; anxiety or guilt arising from previous therapies; and the secondary gains accruing to the patient from his/her symptoms. This last point is very interesting in that it hints at a view of ambivalence which could be considered congruent with behavioral theory. If patients derive secondary gains from their symptoms, a rational explanation for resistance to change is possible.

Even given these examples, it must be said that at least until recently, most behavioral therapists have not dealt with the issue of resistant patients. Their failure to do so is variously explained as a tendency to write about successes, not failures (Hersen, 1971), or the lack of a specific classification of resistances which would stimulate empirical studies, the backbone of the behavioral literature (Jahn & Lichstein, 1980). At least one author has stated that their failure to deal with resistance can be attributed to their lack of analytic training (D'Alessio, 1968), implying that behaviorists have no explanation of their own regarding the phenomenon of resistance. Some have pointed out that behaviorists have spent so little time studying resistance because it is not congruent with their notions of what sustains human behavior, namely, that patients are rational beings, who, given the proper set of contingencies, will change. When patients refuse to engage in behaviors that would ameliorate their stated complaints, they seem irrational. Most behaviorists would be hard put to explain the response of one of our patients who, on being offered a behavioral regimen to help her cope with her stated wish to stop binge eating, said, "This won't work because I know I won't do it."

Resistance, then, "makes the behavioral therapist directly confront his learning theory assumptions concerning the acquisition and maintenance of behavior. The resistive client directly defies the contingencies set by the therapist, and the regulation of behavior via contingency management is a basic tenet of behavior theory" (Jahn & Lichstein, 1980, p. 300). Since resistant behavior makes no sense from a behavioral point of view, it is not surprising that a common behavioral explanation for such situations is that the therapist has failed to discover the correct contingencies. Therefore, it would appear that for most behaviorists the issue would not be one of resistance but of an absence of available reinforcers or insufficient competence on the part of therapists (Hersen, 1979).

Another form of brief treatment which can be described as belonging to the social learning tradition is that of cognitive therapy. This therapy emphasizes teaching patients to think about and perceive their current reality differently. In cognitive therapy, therapists essentially challenge the patient's selective perception of the world by examining the evidence the patient uses to make judgments about self or environment. Cognitive therapists seem to conceptualize resistance as "negative cognitions" about therapy. They suggest that therapists must pay close attention to the patient's self-statements about therapy, attending carefully to such comments as "this won't work" or "therapy has never helped before." To avoid the development of noncompliant behaviors, the therapist refutes such statements and replaces them with more positive attitudes about therapy. Although these prescriptions are clearly designed to avoid resistance, in their popular book *Cognitive Therapy of Depression* (1979), Beck and his colleagues do not specifically address themselves to the issue and, in fact, the word resistance does not even appear in the index. However, the emphasis placed on the establishment of a therapeutic alliance would suggest the importance of such an alliance as a major factor in avoiding resistance. These authors state that the cognitive therapist must be a good psychotherapist, capable of responding to the patient with concern, empathy, and acceptance and "skillful in dealing with transference reaction" (Beck, Rush, Shaw, & Emery, 1979).

The establishment of a collaborative relationship, one in which the therapist actively engages the patient and structures the therapy, but in which the patient carries out much of the work of therapy between sessions, probably avoids resistance. Also probably to avoid noncompliance, or what Mahoney described as countercontrol, Beck and his associates tend to prefer that clients define their own tasks and homework. Further, the therapist, in advance, emphasizes the importance of the client's independent work outside the sessions. Beck *et al.* state, "The patient is encouraged to view homework as an *integral, vital component* of treatment. Homework is not just an elective, adjunct procedure. The therapist usually spends time presenting the rationale for each assignment. The importance of carrying out each assignment is stressed frequently throughout treatment" (Beck *et al.,* 1979, pp. 272–273). Again, to avoid noncompliance, these authors stress the importance of anticipating potential sources of noncompliance with the patient. The emphasis on empathy, acceptance, careful endoctrination, and anticipation of problems with compliance imply that without it, the therapist will fail to engage the patient and the therapy will fail.

Family therapy: In search of a theory of resistance

While the analytic concept of resistance was specifically related to therapists trying to bring about internal change by increasing the insight of one motivated individual, variations on the concept of resistance seem to have survived the transition from classical analysis to most other models of treatment, even those with radically different theories of dysfunction and strategies of change. There appears to be almost universal recognition that resistance exists, if not universal agreement about what to call it, what it is, and what responsibility a therapist has for doing something about it. The field of family therapy includes theorists from both the psychoanalytic and the social learning traditions, as well as theorists who have introduced entirely new concepts. One could expect it, therefore, to contain the same lack of consensus about the existence and nature of resistance that is present in the wider field of psychotherapy, as well as the same lack of agreement on how much responsibility a therapist has for dealing with resistance and bringing about change. Until recently, family therapists have tended to address the issue of resistance indirectly, describing techniques to bring about change which imply that resistance exists and must be overcome without ever explicitly addressing the topic.[1]

The family therapy movement began back in the 1950s, an era when the field of psychotherapy was dominated by psychoanalytic views. A few brave souls who had been trained in preexisting therapeutic traditions, such as the psychodynamic and behavioral approaches, began to focus on the relationship between an individual's symptomatology and his/her current relationships by incorporating ideas from nontraditional sources such as communication, cybernetics, and general systems theory.

Schools of family therapy grew up around these "founding fathers and mothers" who came to hold what is called a "family systems orientation" but who often did not agree on much beyond the basic idea that the family is a system and that behavior can best be understood in the context of the system in which it occurs. Having a "family systems orientation to therapy" describes a general perspective but does little to explain any given school's underlying theoretical assumptions, or philosophy of intervention, much less their ideas about resistance. In fact, family therapists differ so radically from one another that it brings to mind the maxim "In Mexico, everyone is Catholic, including the Protestants."

The lack of clear statements about resistance in most schools of family therapy seems to be related to two issues: the iconoclastic nature of the family therapy movement, and the difficulty in translating the original concept of resistance into a concept relevant to the treatment of family systems. Like any emerging movement, the field of family therapy attempted to establish its boundaries by defining and emphasizing its differences with other existing psychotherapeutic traditions. There is no question that these differences were then and are today significant ones. Early family therapists developed radically different views about what constituted pa-

---

1. The bibliography includes such notable exceptions to this generalization as Hoffman, Stanton, and Solomon.

thology, how to create change, and what the nature of the therapeutic relationship ought to be. The focus of therapy moved from the psychological processes within a patient to the interactional processes within a family. Families were seen as self-governing systems with discernible rules and repetitive patterns of interaction, and symptomatic behavior was redefined as an expression of dysfunction of the family system.

While some schools of family therapy retained an interest in intrapsychic processes, others went so far as to label individual psychopathology, insight, and even historical information as irrelevant in a present oriented conceptual world populated by such notions as hierarchies and feedback loops. In fact, in the course of defining this new territory, some influential pioneers appear to have been almost as interested in attacking and rejecting the cherished beliefs of the psychoanalytic establishment as in developing a new approach to the alleviation of symptoms. The concept of resistance was one of the temporary casualties; it was central to psychoanalysis and therefore had no place in the brave new world of family therapy.

There were other reasons for the rejection of the concept of resistance early in the history of the family therapy movement. In addition to the desire to establish an identity different from that of the reigning psychoanalytic establishment, some of the more radical family theorists claimed there was no need to uncover unconscious, unacceptable thoughts and impulses in order to cause change. This left them without a theoretical framework on which to hang the traditional notion of resistance. Clearly, it was not possible to make an isomorphic translation of the analytic concept to the language of family therapy.

The positions various models of family therapy have taken toward the issue of resistance vary, but not necessarily according to how they view the importance of internal processes. Schools of family therapy can be seen as existing on a continuum between the psychodynamic and object relations therapists, who value intrapsychic processes almost as much as their analytic colleagues, to the Mental Research Institute (MRI) group who take a "black-box" approach and are interested only in observable behaviors. It is interesting that theorists at both ends of this continuum regard resistance as highly significant and take explicit and clear positions on it. On one end of the continuum, Boszormenyi-Nagy and Ulrich (1981) describe resistance in classic analytic terms:

> There is no less resistance encountered here than in the psychoanalytic approach. Avoidance, denial, repression, disassociation, withdrawal, evasiveness, disengagement, failing to face or connect, escape from accountability — by whatever label they are called, these old familiar processes are hard at work in the context of exploring loyalty and legacy. (p. 184)

On the other end of the continuum, Watzlawick says,

> Resistance is very important. Once you learn to use it, you really have come to

a point where you can be effective. To concentrate only on positive things, to my mind, makes for a very ineffective therapy. Resistance is a far more important therapeutic issue. (cited in Ard, 1982, p. 3)

Resistance is both less explicit and less central among other schools of family therapy. In fact, Whitaker and Keith have stated, "We have trouble with the concept of resistance. It implies the therapist ought to do something about it" (Whitaker & Keith, 1981, p. 214). Nevertheless, a general review of the stance taken by some of the major representatives of family therapy on the topic of resistance may be useful as a background for therapists developing their own approach to dealing with resistance.

The following is a brief review of some of the major approaches to family therapy and the apparent positions taken on resistance.[2] The authors take responsibility for the classification of various therapists into specific categories, and acknowledge that many of the classifications and interpretations of positions may not be acceptable to those so classified. This is particularly a problem for therapists who seem to have evolved from one category to another over the years, and who clearly use more than one theory or method simultaneously.

Psychoanalytic or object relations approaches

The psychodynamic models of family therapy described here are those that attempt to integrate ideas from psychoanalytic and object relations theory with principles of family systems. Included in this group are such family therapists as Nathan Ackerman, Norman Paul, A. C. Robin Skynner, Clifford Sager, Helm Stierlin, and Henry Dicks. What distinguishes this group of therapists is their respect for the influence of historical family processes, in particular early object relations, on individual development and thus on the current relationships established and maintained by individuals. Family pathology generally is viewed as the result of a developmental failure in the family of origin, leaving individuals with unconscious inappropriate expectations regarding the behaviors of self and others which they project onto their current family relationships in the real world. These projective systems are experienced not as internal processes projected outward, but as reality. In other words, behaviors and expectations learned in past relationships are unresolved and inappropriately and unconsciously applied to present relationships. Spouses or parents may attempt to externalize, relive, or master conflicts from their family of origin in their current nuclear family. Symptoms are thought to arise when the intensity of denied emotions and experiences increases sufficiently to threaten the defenses of a family member. Some aspect of internal conflict is then projected onto another family member, perpetuating pathology

2. Detailed reviews of family therapy approaches are available. See, for instance, Barker (1981); Gurman and Kniskern (1981); Walsh (1982).

(Skynner, 1981). Thus, a symptomatic member serves an intrapsychic function for others in the family (Ackerman, 1970). Events from the past, particularly unresolved mourning for past losses, are also thought to affect family members' current abilities to tolerate both separateness and intimacy (Paul & Paul, 1975).

In the psychoanalytic approaches to family treatment, change is viewed as being made possible by helping family members to face and surmount these unfinished developmental tasks. Therapists may do so in various ways: Norman Paul, for instance, stresses the need to relive the experience of unmourned losses (Paul & Grosser, 1965). A. C. Robin Skynner (1981) stresses the use of interpretation and normalization of dynamic processes by identifying projective systems and bringing projected conflicts back to where they belong (within the individual or within the marital relationship), to aid in a more constructive resolution which does not require any family member to be dysfunctional. Like many dynamically oriented therapists, Skynner emphasizes a fairly consistent dynamic explanation of pathology and behavior, but appears to condone a wide variety of methods of intervention. For example, he suggests that denials and distortions can be decreased by direct teaching of new relationship skills or by changing the family power structure (à la Minuchin, 1974a, or Bowen, 1978). Likewise, the role of the therapist can vary from authoritarian and directive, neutral and observing, to that of an equal participant with metacommunicative abilities (Skynner, 1981).

In the psychodynamic approach to family therapy, resistance is viewed as the result of layers of defenses created to avoid reencountering the pain of unfinished early experiences and/or as the result of unrealistic desires for unattainable perpetual gratification. To cope with resistance, Skynner stresses the need for therapists to use an awareness of the feelings stimulated in them by the family (be these sexual feelings, tension, or preoccupation) to understand underlying family dynamics. It is assumed that these feelings in the therapist are caused by the denied feelings or issues of the family. After developing trust, therefore, therapists share their feelings with family members, thus normalizing the family's own feelings and decreasing the need to resist (Skynner, 1981). To cope with resistance to reclaiming feelings in the process of operational mourning, Normal Paul uses dramatic evocative techniques, including life-size photographs of the lost person, and tasks, such as visiting gravesites. These techniques are assumed to release and make available denied and defended feelings.

Three-generational approaches

Murray Bowen, Ivan Boszormenyi-Nagy, and James Framo are perhaps the most well-known advocates of approaches which can be classified as three-generational (Gurman & Kniskern, 1981). Murray Bowen, in particular, has accumulated a large following of therapists, many of whom have added their own special permutations to the method (Guerin, 1976; Fogarty, 1976; Friedman, 1971; Carter & McGoldrick, 1980; Kerr, 1981; etc.) Each of the three main proponents has a psychoanalytic background, although this is not usually explicitly acknowledged. While each of these therapists has developed his/her own theory and technique of family intervention, there are some common elements. In each approach, pathology in current family relationships is viewed as related to unfinished business in family of origin relationships (Framo, 1981; Bowen, 1978; Boszormenyi-Nagy & Spark, 1973). Assessment and intervention focus on an exploration of transgenerational patterns (Walsh, in press).

For Murray Bowen, the goal of therapy is the increased differentiation of individuals within families. He attempts to decrease individual anxiety and emotional reactivity so that people can think straight and avoid the need for triangulation or emotional cutoffs which he views as occurring when anxiety becomes high. He generally works with couples rather than whole families, encouraging spouses to work on their relationship with their family of origin.

Ivan Boszormenyi-Nagy (Boszormenyi-Nagy & Spark, 1973) also encourages a reencounter with one's family of origin but stresses a somewhat different purpose. Since he views loyalty as the central motivating factor in life, he believes health is achieved through creating a balance of forces toward repayment or loyalty to family and self-fulfillment. Healing past stagnant or unfinished relationships is thought to improve present ones.

While James Framo does not stress differentiation or loyalty to the degree that the previously mentioned authors do, he does hypothesize that current family and marital problems are caused largely by attempts to master early family-of-origin conflicts (Framo, 1981). He views the problems of children as metaphors of the quality of the marital relationship, which in turn is a function of each partner's unresolved family of origin conflicts. Framo differs from Bowen (1978) and Boszormenyi-Nagy (Boszormenyi-Nagy & Ulrich, 1981) in that he actually seeks to involve members of the family of origin in therapy sessions. In all three cases, however, attempts are made to detriangulate the past (to remove it as a force in current behavior) in order that individuals may better deal with the present.

These authors differ greatly in terms of dealing with resistance. Boszormenyi-Nagy (Boszormenyi-Nagy & Ulrich, 1981) has the most traditional view, seeing resistance as an integral part of treatment and essentially implying that the process of working through resistance is central to its resolution. Framo (1981) also sees resistance as inevitable and indicative of the potential power inherent in a three-generational approach. He, however, places less emphasis on working through resistance and describes techniques which seem designed to minimize it. He carefully prepares family members for such techniques as sessions with their family of origin, and talks of therapists using themselves as models, emphasizing their own life experience to help family members to have the courage to experience the pain inherent in therapy. He does, in other words, take responsibility for making therapy palatable to families and for coping with their resistance.

Bowen (1978), on the other hand, is very clear that he does not view himself as responsible for getting patients to accept, begin, or continue therapy. Based on the assumption that unresolved issues with a family of origin affect current relationships, therapy constitutes a cognitive reencounter with the past as it is represented in the present. In this model of therapy, individuals must reenter their families and rework their relationships with significant primary individuals. The goal, however, is not to change others in the family, but to change the way the focal individual perceives and copes with them. For Bowen, family members remain clearly in charge of their own goals and tasks, with the therapist acting as a coach to help them decide how to achieve their goals. If therapists can do this without becoming caught up in the family's "game," they can help families to change themselves. As in traditional psychoanalytic practice, change relies on the motivation of patients to overcome their own resistance. They should either bring their own motivation or they might as well stay home.

Nevertheless, there are several ways in which Bowen (1978) also deals with resistance indirectly, mostly by employing methods which avoid provoking it. First, he attempts to assume an unbiased research attitude while questioning relationships and assumptions, and focuses on patterns and facts, not feelings. By making use of humor, stories, and reversals to encourage family members to see things differently, Bowen avoids power struggles and confrontation. His neutral attitude and indirect style is less likely to stimulate anxiety and thus resistance than more direct approaches. Second, he assesses a system to discover the most likely point of entry (i.e., the person most able to change), thus calculating the leverage of the system, and then concentrating on using that leverage. In other words, he goes with the least resistant member, only later possibly helping that motivated family member to deal with the resistance of other family members. In this way, he avoids resistance and the need to deal with it directly. Finally, his conducting the therapy of one partner in front of another or in front of a multiple family group seems to serve the same function. "Resistant" individuals need only listen to others work; but they may "incidentally" get something for themselves.

Structural approach

The structural approach to family therapy is primarily associated with Salvador Minuchin and his colleagues at the Philadelphia Child Guidance Clinic: Braulio Montalvo, Harry Aponte, and, later, Lee Combrink-Graham, H. Charles Fishman, M. Duncan Stanton, and Thomas

Todd. These therapists are primarily concerned with boundaries, the subsystem patterns of families, the relationships between the subsystems, and the relationship of the entire family system and its wider ecological environment (Barker, 1981). This approach maintains that individual symptoms represent a family's failure to accommodate its structure to the changing environmental and developmental requirements of its members (Walsh, in press). Symptoms are seen as sustained by the operational structure of the family as evidenced by the ways in which family members relate to each other. Dysfunctional sets (non-problem-solving reactions to stress) develop which perpetuate problems (Minuchin, 1974b). "Therefore," state Aponte and Van Deusen (1981), "whatever the history of the problem, the dynamics that maintain it are currently active in the structure of the system, manifesting themselves in the transactional sequences of the family" (p. 315).

Structural therapists place great emphasis on the strength of a family's homeostatic mechanisms which they describe in terms of rules governing how family members interrelate. These rules, viewed as beyond the awareness of family members, must change in order for the family's structure and thus the symptomatic behaviors of family members to change. The responsibility for change is primarily that of the therapist who causes change by employing three main strategies: challenging the symptom, challenging the family structure, and challenging the family reality (Minuchin & Fishman, 1981). To accomplish these tasks, therapists first "join" families; that is, they negotiate the family's boundary in such a way as to be accepted by the family and to be endowed by the family with the power to be therapeutic. This process is one which Minuchin and Fishman liken to that of getting into the family's boat in the role of helmsman (Minuchin & Fishman, 1981). They then encourage the family to transact family business so that they can observe the process and develop hypotheses about the family structure. Repetitive dysfunctional patterns become the target of therapy, with therapists relying on tasks and directives to restructure family transactions.

With the exception of Stanton and his colleagues (1981), structural family therapists do not emphasize resistance per se. However, they clearly assume that families resist change, whether this change is required by changing environmental and developmental needs or by therapists. Minuchin and Fishman flatly state, "During the family's common history, rules that define the relationships of family members to one another have developed. Any challenge to these rules will be countered automatically" (Minuchin & Fishman, 1981, pp. 28–29). While structural family therapists sometimes refer directly to therapists' activating resistance in individual family members, they are more likely to describe resistance as a function of homeostatic mechanisms. The emphasis placed by structural family therapists on "joining" maneuvers, and the careful attention they pay to the way in which tasks and directives are presented can be seen as prescriptions for avoiding, minimizing, or overcoming resistance even if they are not presented as such. These techniques seem based on the assumption that families will resist not only change in general, but the influence of the therapist, an outsider, in particular. Further, the techniques imply that it is the therapist's responsibility to deal with resistance. Consider the following passage which both describes resistance as functioning to maintain the homeostatic balance and underlines the therapist's responsibility for overcoming the resistance:

> Family members have a discriminating sense of hearing, with areas of selective deafness that are regulated by their common history. Furthermore, all families, even those consisting of highly motivated people, operate within a certain range. As a result, the therapist's message may never register, or it may be blunted. The therapist must make the family "hear," and this requires that his message go above the family threshold of deafness. (Minuchin & Fishman, 1981, p. 116)

Structural family therapists, then, while not concerned with either the past or the unconscious, expect resistance and are prepared to deal with it, especially as it is represented by the family's attempts to exclude the therapist or the family's failure to follow directives. Therapists are viewed as responsible for avoiding or overcoming resistance, and are asked to modify their timing, their style, and their interventions to accommodate to what families can use.

Behavioral approaches

Behavioral family and marital therapy is based on the assumption of social learning theory and/or exchange theory that behavior is learned and maintained by contingencies in an individual's social environment. These approaches include such adherents as Gerald R. Patterson, Robert S. Weiss, Neil S. Jacobson, James Alexander, and Richard B. Stuart. Although there are differences between those who practice marital versus family intervention, in general family dysfunction or pathology can be said to exist when family members have failed to learn adequate social skills or have come to reinforce or at least fail to extinguish negative or symptomatic behaviors in other family members. For instance, a child's acting out may be the result of inadequate or inconsistent limit-setting behaviors on the part of its parents, who thus may be unwittingly reinforcing symptomatic behaviors. Marital problems may be the result of poor skills in the areas of communication and/or conflict resolution (Jacobson, 1981), or a preponderance of negative over positive exchanges in family relationships.

The aim of family therapy for those with a behavioral orientation is to teach parents and spouses more effective ways of dealing with one another by changing the interpersonal consequences of their behavior, specifically altering the contingencies of reinforcement. After conducting an assessment which specifies the contingencies maintaining undesirable behavior (the setting in which it occurs, the people present, etc.), therapists clarify specific goals (at times even using written contracts), and then proceed to teach new skills, model new behaviors, and otherwise require new behaviors by assigning tasks and homework.

Like their non-family-oriented colleagues, behavioral family therapists usually do not address the issue of resistance directly. Jacobson and Margolin are an interesting exception in that they mention resistance explicitly, but they do so in order to stress the negative impact of the concept. Arguing that therapists attribute treatment failures to resistance rather than accepting the blame for inadequate treatment methods, they state:

> Resistance to change seems to function . . . as a way of rationalizing unsuccessful treatment. The presumption that couples will resist change has the potentiality of a self-fulfilling prophecy. If therapists expect couples to resist their change efforts, their in-session behavior will be significantly affected, and they are likely to generate resistance. (Jacobson & Margolin, 1979, p. 45)

However, these authors, like many behaviorists, do seem to attend to issues of resistance implicitly by suggesting strategies that will minimize the likelihood that resistance will occur, and maximize the likelihood that therapists will not have to deal with it in the early stages of therapy. For instance, in a book on marital therapy, Jacobson and Margolin (1979) suggest several methods of avoiding resistance. It is avoided by screening couples for suitability, ruling out those where one spouse is having an affair or where one partner doesn't want therapy. During a carefully conducted assessment of the couple's problems, they also emphasize the therapist's responsibility for the "induction of a collaborating set," pointing out that couples rarely enter therapy in a cooperative mood (Jacobson & Margolin, 1979). A collaborative set is at least in part produced by presenting the couple with an analysis of their relationship which implies reciprocal causality and mutual responsibility and stressing the need for a commitment from both spouses. During this assessment, couples are given time to learn about therapy before they are asked to commit themselves to it. In this method, early interviews with couples are structured to emphasize the strengths of the relationship in order to contribute to a positive view of it by the spouses. Presumably resistant couples would drop out in the assessment phase, thereby helping therapists to avoid both resistance and treatment failures.

Strategic family therapy

Strategic family therapy as it was originally developed by the group at the Mental Research Institute (MRI) in Palo Alto was influenced by three major forces: the communication theories of Gregory Bateson (Bateson,

Jackson, & Haley, 1956), the induction and hypnotic processes of Milton Erickson (1954), and the clinical wisdom of Don Jackson (1965). More recently, Haley's strategic views seem to have evolved somewhat differently (1976), and another model of strategic family therapy has been developed by the Milan group, Mara Selvini Palazzoli, Luigi Boscolo, Gianfranco Cecchin, and Giuliana Prata (1978), and replicated and expanded by therapists at the Ackerman Institute in New York (Hoffman, 1981; Papp, 1980, 1981; etc.). The MRI group, perhaps because of its California context, adopts a here-and-now black-box orientation to internal processes (i.e., there is no need to know or understand either past or internal processes). The Milan group, perhaps because of its European tradition, appears to look at symptoms not only in the context of the present, but also in the context of the family's history (Selvini Palazzoli et al., 1978).

Strategic family therapists, like most of their family therapy colleagues, assume that families operate with repetitive sequences of interactions which define the family's unwritten rules. In normal families, the rules are modified as development and circumstances require. In dysfunctional families, the family has been unsuccessful in its efforts to change to meet the changing needs of its members. Changes required by the evolution of the life cycle or the evolution of circumstances have been responded to by coping mechanisms which have been repeated or escalated despite their failure to resolve problems. Families come to treatment not because of the problems themselves, but because they are at an impasse in their attempts to resolve their problems. They not only have been unable to find effective solutions, but strategic therapists assume a family's efforts to solve their problems have come to perpetuate them. Accordingly, families are thought to need therapeutic intervention precisely because they are resistant to change, and strategies designed to produce change seem predicated on the notion that resistance is central and will have to be used creatively to resolve the impasse.

To overcome resistance, strategic family therapists often attempt to change the perceived reality of family members through the use of relabeling and reframing techniques. A therapist, for example, may relabel a particular piece of behavior to alter its meaning in the family context, or may redefine the family situation so that the perceived meaning of a behavior is less negative. Strategic family therapists also heavily rely on the use of paradox which uses the strength of the family's resistance to change in order to move them toward their goals. For example, the most common paradoxical interventions are prescriptions to continue or increase the same sort of behavior the family has come to the therapist to change, unbalancing the stuck system in a sort of therapeutic Kung Fu maneuver. The theory is that prescribing more symptomatic behavior will emphasize that family members can in fact control their symptom. Prescriptions for increasing the symptom are frequently linked with a relabeling of that behavior. The Milan group, for instance, hook the symptom to its function in the family in such a way that the family psychologically "recoils." They then prescribe that the family continue to function in the same way, with the symptom bearer continuing to be dysfunctional because such behaviors are necessary to preserve the family. The idea is that this prescription not to change behavior defined as perpetuating one member's symptoms is so appalling that family members alter their behaviors. Reminiscent of the Yugoslavian proverb "Tell the truth and run," an important part of such interventions is to deliver prescriptions at the end of sessions so that the disequilibrating value of the suggestion is not dissipated by ongoing conversation about the therapist's comments.

Many centers of strategic therapy use a team of observers to maximize the impact and power of interpretations and produce radical change. Obviously such powerful techniques dictate that therapists take an enormous amount of responsibility for change. The strategic therapist's position on the responsibility of therapists has always been extreme. Their position can be illustrated by a statement variously attributed to Haley or Jackson that there are no impossible families, only inept therapists. (Stanton, 1981, however, reports that on at least one occasion, Haley has recommended therapy be postponed because the therapist had no leverage, indicating that even Haley believes there are at least some situations in which families are impossible to treat.) Selvini Palazzoli modifies this extreme position, only taking responsibility for jarring the family loose from its impasse, not for how they will ultimately change. She states, "Our families are clever enough to solve their own problems after I have interrupted their repetitive pattern (game)" (Selvini Palazzoli, 1981).

Although most strategic therapists rely heavily on paradox, Peggy Papp (1981) makes the point that "if motivation is high enough and resistance low enough for a family to respond to direct interventions, such as logical explanations, suggestions or tasks, there is no need to resort to a paradox" (p. 201). Gurman and Kniskern interpret her point to be that the use of paradoxical techniques may have negative effects and, therefore, should only be used where resistance is great (Gurman & Kniskern, 1981).

Lynn Hoffman, an eloquent spokesperson for the family therapy movement in the past, addresses the issue of resistance directly. She acknowledges that resistance does exist, specifically that families make countermoves to the moves of the therapist, and that when threatened with change these countermoves may include escalation of their problems to the point where the therapist becomes frightened and backs off. She also notes that the therapist may become the target of family members' negative affect, accounting for the fact that resistance often feels negative to the therapist (Hoffman, 1981). However, she challenges the usefulness of a concept of resistance which is based on the notion of family homeostasis, a concept she believes is widely held among family therapists. She advocates adopting a new view of resistance: "It is more accurate to describe resistance as the place where the therapist and client or family intersect. Resistance is merely an artifact of that time and place. . . . We can think positively about resistance, since if often generates the momentum needed to accomplish change" (Hoffman, 1981, p. 348). This description has the advantage of clearly labeling resistance as a force in the therapeutic system rather than in the client or family, and as potentially useful in producing change.

These are only examples of how some of the major schools of family therapy approach the concept of resistance. Given the lack of clarity within the field, it is not surprising that some family therapists have chosen to deny the usefulness of the concept (Dell, 1982; Hoffman, 1981) or even to deny that resistance exists at all. Dell (1982), for instance, states, "Species do not resist the environment: they either survive or they do not." Likewise, in a paper proclaiming the "death of resistance," de Shazer (1980) takes the view that there are no resistant families, only misunderstood families. What looks like resistance, he claims, is the family's "unique way of cooperating."

A pragmatic approach to resistance

Tales of my death have been greatly exaggerated.—Mark Twain

Old concepts never die, they just get relabeled and endlessly modified. While relabeling resistance as a family's unique way of cooperating may temporarily diffuse the negative responses of therapists, as in the move from "psychopath" to "sociopath," the new label soon acquires the old connotation. The next generation of family therapists may just be saying "this family has an impossible unique way of cooperating." Clearly, it would be far better if the field of family therapy could develop a coherent theory of resistance which reflected an understanding not only of family systems and how they operate, but also of therapeutic systems, the context in which family therapy takes place. However, considering the current divergence of views in the field, it is unlikely that a coherent theory will be forthcoming. There is too much about resistance that family therapists do not agree about or have not addressed. Do families resist change, resist influence, or both? Do they resist because symptoms serve a function for the system, because they lack the necessary skills, or because they fear the unknown? Is resistance an unconscious process which must be worked through, or a series of behaviors to be avoided, overcome, or used to achieve change? Is the family responsible for overcoming its own resistance, is it the therapist's business to do so, or should this be a shared task?

Since a coherent theory of resistance is currently out of the question, family therapists must learn to use an operational, pragmatic view which regards resistance as a natural and universal phenomenon, a kind of therapeutic fact of life. Not only is it inevitable that families will resist change, but it is also inevitable that therapists new to the family systems approach will resist learning it, and institutions heavily involved in other models of intervention will resist supporting it. Therapists who can gain an understanding of why resistance is inevitable and how to deal with it in families, agencies, and themselves will find they can see more families more successfully.

A working definition

Resistance can be defined as all those behaviors in the therapeutic system which interact to prevent the therapeutic system from achieving the family's goals for therapy. The therapeutic system includes family members, the therapist, and the context in which the therapy takes place, that is, the agency or institution in which it occurs. Resistance is most likely to be successful, that is, to result in the termination or failure of family therapy, when resistances are present and interacting synergistically in all three components of the therapeutic system.

While it may not be strictly accurate to label all behaviors which impede family therapy as resistance, functionally they operate as resistance and thus deserve to be a part of a pragmatic view. For example, consider the following hypothetical case: A young couple experiencing marital problems struggle with their ambivalence about asking for help. They finally decide that they must seek counseling or their marriage will fail. They don't know where to turn, but after a few phone calls they are directed to their local mental health center. There they discover that they must each go through a standardized intake interview consisting mostly of questions about their mood, their mental status, and their physical and mental health history. Furthermore, they must also submit to a financial interview to determine whether they are eligible to use the agency's services. They find this process embarrassing and irrelevant. When they are finally referred to the appropriate clinician for marital therapy, they are irritable. How well the therapist understands and responds to what they have gone through to reach him/her will determine whether they ever make it beyond the phone call to the first therapy session. Should the family therapist be put off by their expressions of irritation at the system, becoming defensive, rigid, or impatient, he/she may provide the coup de grace which discourages them from coming at all. Abrupt explanations of the system's rules, failure to offer convenient appointment times, or premature interpretations of their "resistance" may terminate contact between helping system and family. In this example, resistance can be seen to arise from an interaction of three parts of the therapeutic system; the family, the therapist, and the service delivery system. While behaviors in these components always interact, for purposes of discussion, the authors will arbitrarily divide these three types of resistance into family based, therapist based, and institution based.

Family-based resistance: Why families resist change

Family therapists make two basic assumptions which are important to a theory of resistance: First, the ways in which families operate are determined by a combination of the heritage brought from each parent's family of origin, and the way in which the inevitable differences between husband and wife have been dealt with throughout the history of their relationship. Second, that families organize themselves in ways which reinforce the identities of their individual members and which insure the survival of the family as a unit. Both these assumptions go a long way toward an understanding of why families resist change.

The heritage each spouse brings to a new marriage contributes to the development of patterns of relating that become habitual over time. Old habits are *diablos conocidos,* that is, known devils. They are deeply embedded in the myths, values, and belief systems which people internalize in childhood. Habits of relating, even those which are not quite satisfactory to family members have the advantage of being familiar and have a history of consequences which are predictable and safe. Most people accept such ways of relating as basic assumptions about life and are largely unaware of the expectations and standards by which they evaluate the behaviors, attitudes, and role performances of other family members (Reiss & Oliveri, 1980). Habitual patterns provide family members with a sense of security, predictability, and a sense that they are acting "right." A comment such as "a wife should handle the family budget" indicates a belief about role behaviors and how things should be managed in a family which is probably based on how things were managed in the individual's family of origin. Change is unlikely, because loyalty to the values of one's family of origin combine with the fact that such beliefs remain unexamined, unless a situation arises in which someone questions "why" a wife should do so. The reasons families behave as they do usually include a number of such unexamined beliefs about relationship management and role behaviors. These beliefs lead us all to attribute meanings to behavior which become powerful regulators of a family's emotional life and its patterns of interaction. In a sense, individual expectations come to define and create interpersonal experience. Beliefs such as "a family should always be close" or "people who love each other never get angry with each other" can take on the power of rules of relating, with potentially dire consequences if they are broken.

It is easy to understand why people resist changing their habits of relating, as the saying goes, "better a known devil than an unknown saint."

The prospect of change in intimate personal relationships is more threatening to an individual's sense of emotional security than most other changes. It is not surprising that most people respond with fear and resistance. Change is frightening and could result in a situation that is worse than the current one. Loss of one sort or another always accompanies change. In order to change, individuals must give up something valued or thought to be essential, often giving up reality as they see it.

The result is that families sometimes cling to familiar behavior patterns to the extent that they are unable to make the changes necessary to promote the growth of their members or to resolve problems in a creative way. Their habits and fears limit their perception of the alternatives open to them. For example, a young mother of three was referred for family therapy with the presenting complaint of severe anxiety attacks. This woman operated under the belief that good wives never criticize their husbands, a belief she acquired unconsciously from observing her mother's behavior, and one which was reinforced by her husband's angry defensiveness when she did venture mild criticism in the early days of their marriage. She felt it was her duty not to criticize her husband even though she disapproved of the harsh way in which he disciplined their children. She said nothing, but consistently compensated for his behavior by being extremely lenient with them. He responded by becoming more strict, and thus a circular, self-perpetuating, and escalating pattern of parenting was established. This young woman became increasingly anxious as financial problems exacerbated the already growing tension in their home. She felt that if she said anything about her husband's irritability with the children, she would merely add to the burdens under which he was struggling, burdens which she feared might lead him to abandon his family. Soon she was making trips to the emergency room, overwhelmed with anxiety and convinced she was going to die. It was only when a therapist included her family in her ongoing therapy that her fear of criticizing her husband and their differences over disciplining their children emerged. With the therapist's help, she was able to voice some of her concerns and was surprised to find that, far from reacting unfavorably, her husband was eager to negotiate a change in their behavior toward the children. He had been increasingly frustrated by his inability to make simple rules stick, unaware that his wife had been tacitly ignoring these rules. They were able to negotiate some mutually acceptable guidelines for managing the children, and the experience of dealing with each other cooperatively went a long way to decrease this wife's anxiety about her marriage and increase her confidence in herself.

The behavior patterns of any family are also reinforced by a family's myths about each other and their own special notions about their historical development. For example, a man may say, "My wife and I are so different. I've always been a person who likes to touch and be touched whereas my wife prefers not to be touched." What both he and his wife may have forgotten is that when they were first married she liked to be touched, but that over the years the husband's inability to differentiate between when she desired affection and when she desired sex, and the wife's inability to talk about this topic, had caused her to avoid touching whenever she did not want sex so that she could avoid sending the wrong message. Whether she was too shy to tell her husband that he was mistaking her need for affection with her need for sex, or whether she had not consciously made the distinction herself, over the years, the myth about their natures had been invented to "explain" their behavior. Both husband and wife resist changing this myth as they have accepted it as a perhaps immutable truth.

While all families operate according to unconscious rules which are the result of how they have worked out the inevitable differences between marital partners, some families seem to be organized in such a way that one member's symptoms either obscure problems in another part of the family or prevent such problems from occurring. In other words, one member's symptoms seem to serve a purpose in assuring the continuation of the family unit. To return to the young mother with anxiety attacks, it can be hypothesized that those frightening symptoms masked her unexpressed anger toward her husband, an anger she believed had the potential to cause the dissolution of the marriage if she expressed it directly. It was actually easier to tolerate the constant fear of death than to tolerate the fear of being assertive or being disloyal to her husband which might result in her being abandoned.

Human loyalty to the family group probably began as a survival strategy long before our ancestors could articulate such a sophisticated concept. Membership in a primary group assured a share in the spoils of the hunt and protection from predators. To survive, these groups had to develop clear boundaries to distinguish who belonged and who might be a potential foe.

While families no longer guarantee survival in the primitive sense in which they did for the millions of years before agriculture was developed and stationary societies appeared, the family's role in insuring psychological survival is nearly as powerful. Humans may almost be said to be genetically programmed to be loyal to their primary groups. As Boszormenyi-Nagy and Spark (1973) emphasize, no therapist can afford to ignore the powerful force of family loyalty.

Families serve to define and maintain the self-concepts of their members. It is natural that family members will resist changing patterns of relating which are central to their sense of personal identity. For example, Joanie, an overly dependent young woman in her 20s declared openly in a family session that if she stopped being so dependent on her parents, she would have no relationship with them at all. In her perception, her sense of self was as her mother's daughter and her mother's definition of self was of self-as-mother-of-Joanie. The thought of changing their relationship to one of more equality and psychological distance brought the threat of mortally wounding herself and her mother and dissolving the family. She could not conceive of how she could emancipate herself without destroying her loved ones.

The constancy of change

While families tend to resist change, they are, of course, required to deal with it all the time. In addition to homeostatic mechanisms, families also have morphogenic ones (Speer, 1970). The tasks of marital sexuality and companionship, the bearing and raising of children, the weathering of crises imposed from the outside environment, or the changing needs of family members all require that a family be able to change while still maintaining a sense of family identity and stability. The forces for and against change must exist in what Lyman Wynne (1980) has called a "dynamic equilibrium." If the forces that resist change are too weak, the family is faced with constant chaos and disruption. If the forces that resist change become too strong, families rigidly fail to adapt to the changing needs of their members. Most family therapists would agree that such families develop what Minuchin calls "stereotyped functioning" (Minuchin, 1974a), a rigid set of acceptable behaviors which thwart individual growth. These rigid behaviors are governed by rules of which families are usually unaware. For example, the parents of our aforementioned Joanie were unaware that they behaved in ways which discouraged Joanie's psychological growth. Her mother had made Joanie her best friend and confidante. Both of them functioned as if they were Joanie's father's children, constantly acquiesing to his bid to control their behavior and dictate their attitudes. As Joanie progressed through adolescence, neither of her parents was able to make the changes necessary to allow her to withdraw her dependency on them and invest her energies in her peers. By the time she was 21, Joanie was withdrawn and devoid of social skills, terrified of risking rejection by trying to make friends. She became a prisoner in her own home, clinging to her parents as her only source of nurturance and stability.

It can be speculated that Joanie's mother may have felt, but not expressed, resentment of her husband's excessive control. This resentment may have gone underground because she had learned in her family of origin that criticism was not acceptable, and/or because her husband's response to her efforts to deal directly with the issue in the early years of the marriage led her to believe that the marriage would be endangered if she continued in this manner. Whatever the reasons, the result was that Joanie and her mother came to function as a dyad, covertly resisting their spouse/parent, a dyad which constricted Joanie's opportunities to explore relationships outside the family. Since her emancipation might have threatened the survival of the parental unit, her parents were quite content to allow Joanie to remain a child in their home. It was only when Joanie began to engage in obsessive rituals that they sought help.

Whatever the causes, the need for stability in families is so strong that it is usually not the desire for change that leads families to seek therapy, but rather it is the *failure* to accommodate to change. Most families come to therapy in *response to changes* which they do not like or have not adjusted to. The sequence of change and therapy is not unlike the sequence noted by Eric Hoffer when he suggests that revolutions do not occur to accomplish change, but rather in response to it:

> Actually, it is drastic change which sets the stage for revolution. The revolutionary mood and temperance is generated by the irritations, difficulties, hungers, and frustrations inherent in the realization of drastic change. Where things have not changed at all, there is the least likelihood of revolution. (Hoffer, 1963, p. 6)

Most families come to therapists to restore stability that has been threatened. Whether caused by the inevitable progression of the life cycle or events experienced individually by family members, most families come for help when they must adjust to something new, and are having trouble doing so (Carter & McGoldrick, 1980; Hadley, Jacob, Milliones, Caplan, & Spitz, 1974). It is natural, therefore, that they should resist the therapist's efforts to change things even more. Therapists who assume that families are unambivalently seeking change will be insensitive to the problems a family has accepting therapy, and may alienate families by moving too quickly or in the wrong direction. A family may come because a shaky parental/marital coalition is having difficulty withstanding the demands for consistency of an acting-out adolescent. In requesting therapy, such parents are probably really hoping that the therapist will somehow transform their sullen, angry adolescent back into the sweet child he/she used to be, rather than asking them to learn to allow his/her awkward attempts toward emancipation. Similarly, a wife who brings her unfaithful husband to therapy may want the therapist to help stop his infidelity. She may not be at all interested in changing the nature of their marital relationship.

Family-based resistance: Why families resist therapeutic influence

Individuals and families, which are after all collections of individuals, not only resist change, but also have negative reactions to any external attempt to influence them. Since we were two years old and learned to say no to our parents, most of us have been busy asserting our own will and attempting to avoid the undue influence of others. In our society, to allow oneself to be influenced is to give away one's fundamental right to self-determination, one's constitutional right to make decisions. Entering any form of psychotherapy constitutes the formation of a dependent relationship and therefore a loss of personal freedom.

Even if families do not assume therapists are going to take over and tell them what to do, the mere selection of a therapist places family members in the position of being vulnerable to the perceived reality, value judgments, and skills of a relative stranger. For example, the antagonistic businessman who called to request help in curing his daughter's anorexia was reacting in part out of a fear of losing his personal freedom and forming a dependent relationship. He owned his own company and was used to exercising a great deal of control over those around him. The thought of giving over some of this control to anyone, much less a female mental health professional, was an anathema to him and he responded accordingly.

In addition to a natural tendency to resist being influenced by someone else, particularly a stranger, entering therapy is often viewed as humiliating because it implies that individuals or families cannot solve their own problems. There is a stigma about not being able to make it on your own. The implication is that if you have the right to live your own life as you see fit, you also have the responsibility to know how to do it successfully.

There is an even greater stigma about therapy or counseling if the help sought is supplied by a mental health facility. People worry about being "crazy," or at least about their friends and associates thinking them so. These worries contribute to the exacerbation of whatever anxieties brought people to therapy in the first place. When anxiety is high, the ability to receive and process information is affected. The tendency to "close down" the reception of new data in a new and threatening situation may look and act like resistance, when it is in fact an adaptive attempt to maintain a sense of self and a sense of control over the environment. Thus, resistance cannot be fully discussed without putting it in the context of the therapeutic relationship and its overt and covert goals. Perhaps patients resist therapists because therapists have failed to convince them that the reality they are offering is better than the one patients already have. Whether the resultant behaviors are described as protective or resistive is largely determined by the point of view of the observer.

The net result of all of these factors is that most individuals are at least ambivalent about seeking therapy, leading them to question the input of therapists and the wisdom of the changes they recommend. Such resistance need not be viewed as a mysterious or pathological phenomenon. Resistance does not mean people enjoy their symptoms or their pain, but simply that they are anxious about therapy or do not enjoy being confronted with the awareness that they have been unable to solve their problems on their own.

This ambivalence about therapy in general is even more difficult for those who are entering family therapy. Most families are at least skeptical about, if not overtly resistant to, the concept of family therapy. The anxiety-producing experience of beginning any kind of therapy becomes complicated by the seemingly illogical request that the entire family come in when the problem clearly resides in one member. Why should the family be seen when it is Johnny who doesn't like school or Mary who is "acting up"? Family therapy doesn't make sense unless you assume the family is to blame for an individual's problems. It is not surprising that family members, particularly parents, either maintain the stance that family therapy is unnecessary *or* become defensive, sensing an implied or explicit criticism on the part of therapists that they are to blame for whatever is going wrong. The recommendation of family therapy contains a metacommunication to family members that they are relevant in the development or perpetuation of the identified patient's problems, a message that actually stimulates guilt and increases anxiety at a time when anxiety is already high. While such a communication may serve positive functions as well, it certainly can contribute to the cause of resistance. If family members feel they will be blamed, it is not surprising that they question the wisdom of discussing painful and sensitive issues in the presence of others in their family who may later use the material against them.

Degrees of resistance

Not all families will display equal resistance to being influenced. The level of resistance in each individual family can usefully be seen as being somewhere on a continuum between compliance and defiance (Papp, 1980; Tennen, Rohrbaugh, Press, & White, 1981). Some families will have a predisposition to follow almost any therapeutic directive (which, of course, in itself may be a sort of covert resistance). Others will have a predisposition to what J. W. Brehm has described as reactance, the tendency to do the opposite of what has been suggested in order to reassert one's sense of self-determination (1972). Many factors probably influence where families fall on this continuum: the degree to which family members see their survival as depending on their family's current organization; the degree to which family members value personal freedom; the degree to which therapy seems to threaten to uncover and reveal to outsiders the family secrets, skeletons, and loyalties. Families may move along the continuum as treatment proceeds. Some families will tend toward more defiance in the early stages of treatment only to be less so once the therapist has become familiar to them. Other families are more likely to be initially compliant, tending toward defiance only after some basic pattern or security is challenged or when threatening changes seem to be occurring.

Systems-based resistance: Enter the family therapist

Therapists are introduced to family therapy in many different ways. Most students of psychiatry, psychology, social work, nursing, and schools of counseling do not receive all their training in family therapy. In fact, usually family therapy is a very small part of their overall training experience. Often therapists have received several years of training in individually oriented therapy before they are introduced to family therapy, and in some cases, therapists have practiced individual psychotherapy for years before they have chosen to train in family work. Such newcomers to family therapy must realize that resistance to family therapy is as natural and normal in beginning family therapists as it is in families. It is important to understand what it is about family therapy that is so different from forms of therapy which treat one individual at a time. Family therapy has expanded the concept of how change occurs, and consequently assumes much greater therapeutic responsibility for bringing about change than most forms of individual treatment. While many forms of therapy involve a focus on observable behavior, family therapy has emphasized the importance of the context in which behaviors occur. The behavior of individuals is now viewed as having significance only within the context of their personal systems, and the whole locus of change has shifted from individuals to the system of intimate relationships in which they live. One result of shifting the locus of change from individuals to systems is a change in the meaning and significance of motivation.

Individual family members may be aware of their intentions while not being aware of the functions of their behavior in the system. For example, the individual consciously intends only to make a joke, unaware that his/her behavior is a response to a rise in the anxiety level of other members of the family, that the joke is an attempt to avoid the possibility of open family conflict, a maneuver which is not only expected, but supported by the entire family. Individuals cannot be expected to completely recognize the rules of the system in which they live, nor can they take full responsibility for changing their own family systems. Family rules operate at a meta-level, beyond the level of individual or family awareness. Individual motivation, therefore, is not the major criteria in determining receptivity to therapy and change. If individual motivation alone cannot be depended upon to bring about change, and there probably is no such a thing as "family motivation," who is to be made responsible for causing change to occur? The response of family therapists to this question has been mixed, but the tendency has been to lay responsibility for change at the therapist's doorstep. Like an ultimate technician or an expert repairperson, the family therapist is asked to observe the system and its malfunctions and intervene to make it function satisfactorily again. The whole image is one of a sort of 20th-century cybernetic magician. It is no wonder that those who decided to become therapists because they like working with people have difficulty warming up to this role.

In fact, it is this issue of therapist responsibility that seems to be most problematic for beginning family therapists. It is not always clear to beginners just what they are responsible for. If therapists are completely responsible for overcoming or eliminating resistance in the service of causing change to occur, do families have the right to reject their efforts? Where does a therapist's responsibility for a family end and a family's right to live their own lives begin? Must families, by coming to treatment, submit themselves to the therapist's goals and methods with no chance to conclude that what he/she has in mind isn't what the family wants or isn't worth the price? Do therapists have the right to define this as resistance? If there are no impossible families, only inept therapists, isn't it implied that therapists should be able to cause change to occur, even when families don't want it? This omnipotent stance would seem to reflect undue grandiosity or excessive narcissism on the part of family therapists. Surely a case can be made for greater mutuality in the process of goal seeking and attaining therapeutic change.

This is not to say that the view of therapists as having responsibility for engaging and influencing resistant families hasn't been a contribution of enormous value. No longer can therapists simply dismiss difficult families as "unmotivated." Family therapists have accepted the responsibility for developing ways of connecting with people who traditionally would never have accepted therapy. For instance, the attention Minuchin (1974a) gives to joining the family system in ways that are syntonic with the family's organization and style has no doubt enabled many families to accept therapy to whom that process might otherwise have seemed alien and frightening. Likewise, even de Shazer's (1982) view of family resistance being the family's "unique way of cooperating" has value in this regard. While anyone who has ever worked with a persistently resistant family will tell you that describing their behavior as "uniquely cooperative" just doesn't do justice to the experience, there are at least two benefits which accrue from this process of relabeling: It highlights the therapist's responsibility for joining with the family on their terms, and it decreases a therapist's tendencies to take resistance personally and thus react to families in a counterproductive manner.

Coming to grips with the issue of responsibility in family therapy is particularly difficult for those who have received their primary training in the psychodynamic model of individual psychotherapy. In order to adapt to the role of the therapist in most approaches to family therapy, such therapists must make a major shift in their implicit *and* explicit behavior. While they have been taught not to take responsibility and not to tell people what to do, now they are told they must take responsibility and be directive. Furthermore, they must do so actively. They cannot follow the initiative of the families by turning things back to them and asking, "How do you feel about that?" They are asked to learn a wide range of interventions that require they be active, and even "manipulative" of family systems. Manipulating family systems effectively requires the use of a confusing blend of traditional ideas about influencing people, that is, forming a therapeutic alliance, examining the function of resistances, while at the same time creating change by employing "tricks" reminiscent of the shamans, such as reframing situations and prescribing symptoms.

Unfortunately, much of the attention at workshops and conferences has been focused on these flashier aspects of creating change. While such interventions are actually among the most sophisticated methods discovered by family therapists to achieve change quickly, to the beginner attending such workshops or conferences, the expert family therapist resembles a modern Merlin, producing the illusion of change with a bag full of tricks. They are often repelled or intimidated by these techniques, seeing them as bordering on the unethical, so mystical that they could never master them, or so easy that they attempt to apply them inappropriately without genuine understanding.

Another problem for both beginners and their more experienced colleagues is that of orthodoxy, that is, a sworn allegiance to one approach to family therapy. Therapists who have trained under the influence of a skilled practitioner in a certain approach may resist seeing the limitations of that approach and may resist experimenting with other approaches as the needs of any given case may dictate. While there are limitations to how many models one can hope to learn sufficiently well to practice competently, it is also true that different families respond to different approaches. Therapists who have several models to draw from have an advantage. In the best of all possible worlds, therapists draw from multiple models to evolve their own approach and avoid the need for orthodoxy altogether. This process has the added advantage of encouraging critical self-evaluation and the use of theory as an evolving guide rather than as dogma. However, the competitive nature of the major schools of family therapy and the absence of efforts to make the commonalities of family systems approaches more obvious rather than more obscure, can make the frustration of therapists seeking to evolve their own approach more acute.

Systems-based resistance: The art of fitting four round pegs into one square hole

The whole notion of thinking in terms of systems is popular beyond the field of family therapy. One would think that in this enlightened atmosphere, it would be relatively easy to persuade service delivery systems to start thinking family systems, but this is often not the case (see Chapter 6). Service delivery systems resist incorporating family therapy for some of the same reasons that families resist change and resist being influenced. Institutions have their own *diablos conocidos,* comfortable assumptions about theoretical positions and familiar ways of operating. Anything new threatens the stability of the old. Administrators and senior clinicians often received their training before family therapy became an accepted treatment modality and before it was routinely incorporated as part of training. Such administrators and senior clinicians have experienced success with their own theoretical models and have faith in them. They are not necessarily going to be eager to let them go in favor of a radically different approach. Institutions dedicated to one theoretical position are particularly susceptible to being threatened by new approaches because change threatens both the formal and informal hierarchies.

Family therapy is not just a new modality, it is a very different way of thinking about symptoms and thinking about change. It speaks a new language, one for which there is no easy translation from individually oriented theories. Therapists who wish to begin doing family therapy in agencies and institutions where it is not an established form of practice will also find some practical problems, such as offices which are designed to accommodate only two people, and forms which fail to ask questions about family relationships.

Often there is little a therapist can do to change his/her agency's policies (other than to get permission to practice family therapy), particularly if the agency is heavily invested in another model of intervention. The important point is for therapists to be aware that systems based resistances exist and can interact with their own ambivalence, and that of families, to make family therapy easy to avoid.

Family therapy "sans charisma": A pragmatic view of therapist responsibility

Most family therapists are intimidated by the image created by experts, on videotape or in family therapy road shows, of the family therapist as a 20th-century cybernetic magician. They feel hopelessly inadequate to create the change such experts seem to accomplish with flamboyant techniques and the power of their charismatic personalities. These experts never seem to encounter serious resistance, or to make short work of it with barely a backward glance. What "front line" family therapists fail to realize is that these experts have few problems with resistance because they have spent years fine-tuning their skills and maximizing the use of their assets and personalities. A Whitaker may use his warmth and magnetism to connect with families and inspire cooperation. A Minuchin may maneuver so skillfully that he must rarely encounter resistance head on. Most of us would love to emulate these experts, but lack the charisma and the skill to duplicate their interventions effectively. This does not mean that all family therapists, even beginners, cannot be effective. Although it may seem sacriligous, it is possible to do family therapy without mega-doses of charisma. To do so, however, therapists must become expert in the detection and mastery of resistance. With the ability to recognize resistance and its functions in families, therapists can respond positively and effectively, avoiding, overcoming, or even using resistance as a vehicle for change.

The first step family therapists must take to master resistance is to decide for themselves the question of how much responsibility for change they can take realistically. This decision should be tempered by an awareness of the results of psychotherapy outcome studies which indicate that a good portion of outcome variance is attributable to patient, not therapist, factors (Garfield, 1971). Otherwise, less experienced therapists may be tempted to give up altogether when senior folk suggest that there are no impossible families, only inept therapists. In deciding how much responsibility to assume, family therapists should remember that those who accept complete responsibility for creating change in families are setting themselves up for failure and demoralization. The situation is not unlike that faced by sex therapists following the outstanding success rates published by Masters and Johnson (1970). No one could match their success rates, and many therapists became demoralized, forgetting that Masters and Johnson had elaborate screening procedures and could afford to work with only those clients who were so motivated to deal with their sex lives that they were willing to spend several thousand dollars and two weeks in St. Louis. Most sex therapists have a responsibility to provide service to a community, or need patients in a private practice, and do not have the luxury of screening or refusing difficult clients.

Similarly, most family therapists, unless they are in private practice, have little control over which families they must accept for treatment, as they have a responsibility to provide service to those who request help in their community. Most family therapists are not magicians nor are they in a position to operate as a team, combining the wisdom, insight, and support of a group of colleagues to create strategies for producing change in difficult families. The authors wish to take nothing away from those who are fortunate enough to practice in those institutes where therapists do practice in groups, where they are able to observe each other, and give immediate consultation and support. These therapists and groups perform the important function of developing theories and strategies the rest of us can then use in less ideal surroundings. Nevertheless, a note of realism about the conditions under which most people practice family therapy will help other therapists, particularly beginners, to decide the question of how much responsibility they can take for change in a balanced and realistic way. There are families which have proved themselves resistant to the efforts of many therapists and agencies to bring about change, there are therapists who cannot treat certain families, and there are agencies and institutions which often are not therapeutic because of their administrative structures or their roles in society.

Based on the view that both families and therapists have responsibility for inducing family change, this book will stress the importance of mutual responsibility in the process of facilitating change and overcoming resistance. Therapists will be viewed as having the responsibility for understanding resistance and why it occurs. They also will be viewed as having the responsibility to develop skills for connecting with a wide variety of families, dealing with the resistances they bring, and for understanding and working with their own resistances and those of the system in which they work. This does *not* mean that therapists should have the sole responsibility for creating change or for overcoming all resistance. Therapists who take complete responsibility are destined to be engaged in ongoing struggles in which they push and coax while the family drags its many feet.

On the other hand, therapists should not give sole responsibility for change and resistance to families. Families must be allowed to choose their own goals and to refuse those imposed upon them unilaterally. The authors of this book take the position that a therapist's responsibility to any family is akin to that of a navigator to the captain of a ship. The captain maintains control over the destination of the ship and the idiosyncracies of how it functions. The navigator, however, has the responsibility to use a particular type of knowledge and skill to advise the captain of the best way to reach the ship's destination. If a captain insists on sailing into dangerous waters, a navigator has the responsibility to advise a safer and more effective course to help the ship to reach its port. Likewise, by accepting the role of therapist for a family, a therapist accepts a certain amount of responsibility for the outcome of therapy, including a certain amount of responsibility for establishing and maintaining a therapeutic alliance. Though families become temporarily dependent on therapists to help them reach their goals, therapists must always leave families in charge of determining their own fate.

Summary

Resistance has been defined as a property belonging to a therapeutic system which can be expressed by the behavior of any part of that system. The therapeutic system includes family members, the therapist(s), and the agency or institution in which therapists practice. Resistances residing in different parts of the system are seen as operating in a synergistic and fluctuating manner, any or all of which can interfere with the successful initiation or completion of family therapy. Resistances residing in any part of the system can be expressed overtly or covertly, and can move about between family members or between the family system and the therapeutic system over time.

There are many factors which contribute to the resistance exhibited by a family. However, the major sources seem to be a family's natural striving for stability and a family's equally natural, if sometimes irrational, fear of change. Both of these tendencies lead families to cling to their familiar habits of relating to each other, and to respond with ambivalence to the threat of loss of autonomy and control which seems to accompany therapy. Some families are more sensitive to change and to threats of loss of control, each family at any given time existing at a point on a continuum between compliance and defiance.

While resistance is inevitable, it is almost always accompanied by a desire for relief from the distress which brings the family in contact with the agency or institution.

The existence of resistance does not mean that therapists must do something about it. Many minor resistances are best ignored as inevitable inconveniences to be noted but not necessarily responded to overtly, like slow service in a restaurant. When therapists do intervene, their choice of a type of intervention, and whether to attempt to overcome, avoid, or use resistance to produce change will be based on their theoretical orientation and their understanding of where on the compliance/defiance continuum a family or family member is at any given time.

A word of caution: Family therapists are cautioned not to look at their own behavior and that of families with an eye to shouting, "Aha! Resistance!" and launching a plan to eradicate it. Behaviors serve many functions. The same behavior that may be resistance at one point in time may not be resistance at another. Therapists must always evaluate the context of a behavior to determine its function in the family and the therapeutic system.

While the arbitrary nature of the division of resistance as residing in either the family, the therapist, or the larger service delivery system cannot be overemphasized, this division is necessary to discuss the issues intelligently. The bulk of this book will be devoted to discussion of resistances offered by families. Chapter 4 will discuss methods to avoid the resistances produced in therapists by family member's challenges to their competence, and Chapter 6 will discuss resistances offered by therapists and the agencies and institutions in which they practice, as well as resistance produced in families by the agencies from which they seek help.

2. Initial resistances

THE MOCK TURTLE: Will you, won't you, will you, won't you, will you join the dance?—Lewis Carroll

It would be difficult to overstate the importance of the first contacts between a family therapist and a family seeking treatment. In Chapter 1, resistance was defined as stemming from a number of forces, including a system's natural efforts to maintain stability, most people's somewhat irrational fear of change, and their reluctance to give up control over their lives. Given this definition, it is natural to expect resistance to be particularly strong in the beginning of treatment. Therefore, the need to anticipate, recognize, and effectively deal with it is crucial to the process of beginning therapy. If family therapy is viewed as a kind of dance, with the need for complementary movements on the part of family and therapist, it can be seen that, to be effective, a therapist must learn many invitations to the dance, as well as many different rhythms and steps to accommodate the styles of families. As Braulio Montalvo has been quoted as saying, "If you see families, you will dance to many a tune." This chapter will focus on the mastery of the invitation to the dance, and those often clumsy and awkward movements that occur as dancers attempt to join and adjust to one another's movements. In other words, this chapter will focus on factors which could prevent therapy from getting off to a good start, or to any start at all.

As was emphasized in Chapter 1 and will continue to be emphasized throughout this book, all human interaction occurs within a context which helps to explain the meanings of messages or behaviors. Just as repeating a small part of a politician's statement out of context distorts its meaning, seeing the behavior of a family seeking treatment without considering the context of the treatment system can distort our understanding of the meaning of behaviors. The context for any family seeking treatment consists of the referral, their initial contacts with the system, their knowledge about therapy and what to expect, their idiosyncratic style and other reality factors.

The invitation to the dance: Initial contacts between the family and the system

An important part of the context of families seeking treatment, particularly if it is their first experience with any kind of therapy, is the way in which the recommendation of family therapy is made and the way in which the agency, institution, and/or therapist responds to the family's attempts to follow this recommendation. Families do not usually refer themselves to a family therapist. When they do, it means at least one family member has some idea that the family's problems have to do with how they behave toward one another, thinks a family approach is relevant, and has enough clout within the family to persuade other family members to give it a try. If, as is more usual, a family is referred by someone else, the level of family resistance may relate to how well the referral has been made. The best referrals are made by colleagues who believe in family therapy and are able to present families with a clear and convincing case for why it is relevant and potentially useful. In most settings, however, a large proportion of referrals come from professionals who are unclear themselves about why they are sending someone for family treatment. They may be inspired by instinct, the advice of a supervisor, or the simple fact that nothing else has worked. When professionals referring families are unclear about why they are making referrals, they may find it difficult, if not impossible to explain the recommendation to family members in a helpful and convincing way.

The level of family resistance encountered is also affected by the number of steps between a family's impetus to seek help and the moment when they make contact with the family therapist. In general, the more steps in such a process, the more resistance to family therapy a therapist can anticipate. This is a particular problem in large health care systems, where the family therapist is the second or third professional the family has encountered. Usually, the professionals making the initial contacts have focused on one family member who has been evaluated, tested, labeled, treated, and thoroughly identified as the patient. Often it is only when other treatments have not worked or compliance has become a problem that someone recommends family therapy. Depending on how well this was done, family members may feel grateful, supported, and understood, or they may feel blamed for the patient's difficulties. These policies and processes make it more likely that there will be an extended time delay between the family's request for help and the onset of family therapy, not to mention an increased likelihood that someone will have unwittingly offended the family along the way. What comes across to family therapists in their first contacts with family members who have been through this process may sound like resistance, but may really be an expression of the family's confusion and frustration with the system.

Unfamiliarity with therapy

While a certain percentage of the population seems to regard therapy as part of life, as expected as weekly appointments with hairdressers or music teachers, most people know very little about any kind of therapy, much less family therapy. Even when some professional has taken care to explain to them why family therapy is necessary or desirable for their particular problem, family members will probably approach family therapy with a wide variety of questions. For example, the Family Therapy Clinic recently took a call from a woman who had been told that her children were all behavior problems in school. She told us that while the school counselor had recommended family therapy, her sister who was in college had told her she needed a "behaviorist." Although she did not know what a behaviorist was, she expressed disappointment that the therapist was "only" a garden variety family therapist. Only after the therapist explained that the woman's sister had probably been referring to behavior modification techniques, which she could incorporate in her model of family therapy, was the woman willing to make an appointment. A therapist insensitive to this woman's confusion might have mistaken her unfamiliarty with therapy in general as disinterest in or resistance to a family approach.

Family style, culture, and real-life problems

All exchanges between the therapist and the family at any stage in treatment must involve a consideration of the family's general style of relating and its style of relating in times of stress. A family member's initial anxiety, expressed as hostility or transient bravado, may less reflect serious reservations about family therapy than reservations which can be easily resolved with some explanation of what can be expected. Also, since class, race, and cultural differences may affect the style with which a family approaches the therapeutic process, these variables must be considered in assessing the meaning of the family member's behaviors and thus the level of resistance. For instance, middle-class families who are sophisticated about therapy are more likely to be at least superficially cooperative because they feel it is the socially appropriate way to behave. The family's manners or good form may not necessarily represent a genuine measure of the level of cooperation the therapist can expect. Such families may be just as skeptical as families that question the therapist directly or tell the therapist to "bug off."

The same is true for some cultural groups who are very responsive to authority. Since they tend to invest the therapist with the same sort of power they might invest in the clergy, resistance often goes underground. Some other groups, particularly lower socioeconomic groups, may respond with overt hostility because they tend to see the therapist as an extension of those social agencies which exercise unwanted control over their lives. While these resistances are at least overt, they are somewhat harder on a timid therapist.

The therapist will also do well to remember that real-life problems exist which may interfere with the onset of therapy. An assessment of the level of real-life problems contributing to what seems to be resistance will help the therapist to decide on the most appropriate therapeutic response. Therapists should try not to interpret behavior as resistance until they have observed repeated patterns of behaviors that point to this conclusion. After all, as Freud said, sometimes a cigar is just a cigar. Cars do break down, parents do have to work late, children do fail to come home from school. If a family's appointment is genuinely inconvenient, there is no need to interpret their cancellations or lateness when a simple change in appointment time will do. It is generally best to accept the simplest explanation and try the simplest intervention first. Remember, as the saying goes, "When you hear the sound of hoofbeats, think first of horses, not zebras."

The first phone call: Connections

When making the first phone call, it is important to bear in mind the questions inherent in the factors mentioned above:

1. Was the referral source knowledgeable about family therapy and therefore able to explain clearly the reasons for suggesting family therapy and what the family can expect from it?
2. How many steps have intervened between the family's first impetus to seek help and their contact with the family therapist?
3. What has been the family's previous contact with therapy?
4. What impact will the family's culture, style of relating, and current reality have on the chances of successfully launching the therapeutic process?

Most therapists can cite examples of families who never made it past the first phone call, yet few therapists spend much time considering the importance of this call. It seems a mundane routine, too insignificant a focus when time could be spent considering the more interesting issues of circular causality or enmeshment. However, a lack of attention to mundane routines can result in no chance to observe the subtleties of circular causality and enmeshment because the family is lost before treatment begins. Experienced therapists develop methods of dealing with this call effectively, but seldom pass on the nuts and bolts of these hard-won skills. Consequently, each new trainee must rediscover the wheel, usually through his/her own mistakes.

For a number of reasons, a phone call from a family inquiring about family therapy is more complicated than a call to request individual therapy, not least because of the number of individuals that are indirectly involved in the negotiations. Each member of the family has his/her own particular view of the origin and severity of the problem, the role of his/her own behavior and level of motivation to do something about the problem.

When a family member makes the initial call, his/her purpose may not be actually to engage a therapist, but rather to explore the availability of therapy, its costs, requirements, and potential benefits. In other words, the call may serve as a screening interview during which the representative of the family presents the family's view of the problem and evaluates the therapist's response.

Connecting with the caller

Family members calling about therapy tend to feel vulnerable at the time of the initial contact, and are particularly in need of a sense that they will be treated with respect, that their idiosyncracies will be tolerated, and their problems will be listened to thoughtfully. The therapist must take the time to connect with the member representing the family in their quest for help, establishing a contact strong enough to overcome any initial resistance to coming to a strange place to see a strange person, while not becoming so bonded to the one family member who is calling that the therapist's objectivity is forfeit even before the first interview. While the amount of data collected about the problem will depend on the therapist's theoretical orientation, all therapists must assess what it will take to get the family involved and then, through their representative, begin to involve them. Therapists who are pressed for time, and therefore are simply eager to make the appointment, end the call and get on with other business, may fail to make a strong connection. Furthermore, they may appear unsympathetic or even flip.

Assessing the level and location of resistance

Any member of any family has a biased view of what is going on in the family and will unconsciously pass on this bias to anyone with whom he/she discusses the family's problems. Therefore, therapists making the first contact with one family member must be receptive to this person's statement about the problem without committing themselves to it as the system's only truth and reality. Because therapists know nothing about the family, this process of connecting with the family and assessing their resistance is a little like feeling the way in the dark down an unknown passageway. It's never really possible for therapists to know what they will run into next.

Family members who call will have varying levels of motivation as well as varying perspectives of their own involvement in the problem. It would be a mistake to assume that the person who calls is the most motivated. Sometimes the phone call is made by the one who is most suspicious of therapy. Assuming the family member calling accepts the need for therapy, the best way to avoid being co-opted into a biased point of view is to focus on the problems of arranging for the first interview rather than a long discussion of the problems bringing the family to therapy. Therapists should concentrate on all those practical and attitudinal problems which the family member presents as possible barriers to his/her own participation or that of other family members.

Frequently callers locate the source of resistance as somewhere else in the family system, a family member with whom the therapist is not in direct contact. For example, wives point to their husband's unavailability as the cause of scheduling difficulties, or mothers to the reluctance of their adolescent children. Often parents claim that they are quite willing to come, but that the identified patient is reluctant. Even more often parents can see the logic of displaying the family problem, that is, bringing in the identified patient, but are reluctant to bring in their nonsymptomatic children, particularly if these children are at all resistant. This occurs most frequently in families with adolescent and young adult "children" since younger children are usually more willing to be involved and more susceptible to parental directives.

Relatively early in the call, the therapist must check out how the family has been treated by past therapists or other members of the current health care delivery system, including the referral source. If the family has been put off or alienated, the therapist can begin to build a new relationship with them by being sympathetic to what they have been through and stressing how this therapeutic experience will differ. In this process, it is important to avoid criticizing or defending previous therapists. Criticizing colleagues does not inspire confidence, and defending colleagues may simply embroil the therapist in the family's struggle with past therapists or other health care systems.

If the family's past experiences have been positive, it is often possible to build on their relationship with previous professionals. For example, one family member recently called to inquire about family therapy, stating, "Dr. Blender thinks we need family therapy, but I don't think so." Despite her resistance to family therapy, this mother's respect for Dr. Blender's opinion was sufficient to motivate her to at least make the call. Therefore, rather than launching a dissertation on the benefits of family therapy, the therapist used the mother's respect for Dr. Blender's opinion to say, "I know Dr. Blender is a good doctor and I also respect his opinion. I'm not sure why he recommended family therapy but let's get together and give it a try." Alternatively, the therapist could have asked Dr. Blender to use his relationship with the family to persuade them that therapy is necessary rather than trying to do so himself/herself.

Finally, in assessing the level of resistance during a phone call, it is important not to be misled by form. Both overt and covert resistances will be encountered. Overt resistances are relatively easy to recognize and may be manifested by anything from complaints about the lack of parking facilities in the neighborhood of the clinic, to frankly expressed doubts as to the effectiveness of therapy in general and family therapy in particular. Covert resistances, somewhat more difficult to recognize and deal with effectively, range from the simple omission of relevant information, to the complicated phenomena of pseudocooperation in which the family member calling earnestly appears to agree with everything the therapist says, without any intention of following suggestions or even of telling other family members about the call.

The first phone call: Common expressions of resistance

The following section describes some of the most common forms of resistance encountered in the first phone call. These resistances may occur separately, or the whole series may be presented by one family in the space of one 15-minute phone call. The suggestions given may be used in various combinations depending on the strength of the resistance, the setting, and the therapist.

Problem 1. The problem is located in one member

Most families coming to family therapy do not begin by seeking this form of treatment. Usually they were referred because in the judgment of others, family factors have caused, maintained, or exacerbated the dysfunctional behavior of a family member. During the first phone contact, therefore, it is common that the family member calling locates the problem in another family member and is therefore resistant to the idea that there is a need for the family to be involved.

For example, Mrs. Ewing called to say that her 10-year-old son, Phillip, was having trouble. His school complained that he was failing several subjects, bullying other children, and refusing to mind his teachers. According to Mrs. Ewing, testing by a reputable psychologist had revealed that he was above average in intelligence and able to do the work. Both the psychologist who had done the testing and the school had recommended family therapy, a recommendation Mrs. Ewing claimed she really didn't understand. She denied the family had any other problems and rather defensively pointed out that the other children were fine. She asked if it wouldn't be possible for the therapist to see Phillip individually.

SUGGESTIONS

Accept the Family's View of the Problem. In order to make a good connection with the family member making the call, the therapist must empathize with the caller, and one way or another obtain their agreement to bring the family for treatment. To this end it is entirely reasonable to accept the family's view of the problem without attempting to widen the focus at all. There is no point in raising controversial issues over the phone. Therapists have far more leverage once families are in their offices where they have at least an hour of face-to-face contact in which to persuade them that their problem is best treated with family therapy. In the above case, for example, the therapist can accept the mother's view that Phillip is the family's only problem, while adding that it is his/her policy or the clinic's policy to do an assessment which includes the whole family. Labeling this first contact as part of a routine assessment which must include everyone's input in order for the patient's problem and the family's resources to be fully understood, may make the contact less threatening and more acceptable to family members. The therapist can assure the family that participation in a complete assessment will not commit them to a course of family therapy, and that the family will have a chance to give their opinion about any treatment decisions that are to be made. If resistance persists, as a last resort the therapist may ask the family to come "just this once." The family member may be told that the whole family may not be required to come every time, but that for the initial evaluation their contributions and participation are invaluable. A variation on the message that the family is needed in order to do a complete assessment is the message that the request that the family participate is for the benefit of the therapist, such as in "Well, it really would be most helpful to me if everyone came." The key is to agree to anything that will help the therapist, like the traveling salesperson, to get a foot in the door. Later more productive arrangements can be negotiated.

Accept the Family's View of the Problem but Widen the Problem Definition. As we stated earlier, it is best to avoid long discussions of the presenting problem during the initial phone call to avoid being co-opted by the views of one family member. However, at times the insistence that the problem resides in only one member is so strong that the family is unwilling to even consider coming for an assessment unless some explanation is given. In these cases, a strategy which gradually widens the problem definition can be very useful. Beginning by following the general therapeutic principles of empathizing and "hearing out" the complaints of the family, gradually the therapist begins to introduce nonthreatening questions which expand the focus beyond that of the identified patient. To expand the focus, for instance, the therapist may ask questions about the response of other family members to the identified patient's problem, about events that may be indirectly upsetting the patient by causing stress, or about the likelihood of diminished availability of any family member at this time (changes in a parent's job, family finances, pregnancies, siblings leaving for college, etc.). As data about the entire family are gathered, the focus is kept on the identified patient, but ever widening circles are drawn which establish the relevance of other family members to the *patient's* problem.

As the therapist repeatedly connects other family members to the identified patient, be that in positive or negative ways, the therapist builds a case which helps the family to see why they should be included in therapy sessions. When some convincing reason for involving all family members can be put together out of the information a family member has given, the therapist then makes the request for the family's involvement. In the case of Mrs. Ewing, she admitted that Phillip also bullied his two well-functioning younger siblings, and that his older brother was the only one he listened to at home. The therapist began to define the older brother as potentially useful both in gaining Phillip's cooperation, and as a model for and support to the younger siblings who clearly needed some more effective strategies for coping with their brother.

In another family, a mother called to request therapy, stating that her daughter was binge eating and vomiting during her first year in college. While she claimed that she and her husband would be happy to participate in therapy sessions with this daughter, she saw no reason to involve her two older children who had had no problems in school and who were now successfully emancipated. The therapist used these very data as a rationale for involving the identified patient's two older siblings. Since they both had done exceptionally well in school, their experience as successful college students was defined as being of potential use to their sister who was clearly having trouble negotiating her new environment.

Trade on Past Experience. When the caller sees no reason to involve the whole family the experience of the therapist can be emphasized. Presumably, families call therapists because they expect them to be experts, and therefore, they are sometimes quite willing to accept recommendations if they are given authoritatively. This technique includes variations of the phrase "In my experience, it's always better to involve the whole family." Of course, if therapists elect to use this technique, they must be careful to say, "MY EXPERIENCE" rather than "my experience." When therapists have little experience of their own, other sources of authority may be invoked, such as in "Research suggests that this type of problem is best handled by involving the whole family," or "In the past few years, our team has seen over a thousand families, many of them with problems just like yours. We find that. . . . "

Separate Causality and Treatment. One major reason families are resistant to the idea of family therapy is because they believe it implies that they are to blame for the identified patient's troubles. It sometimes helps to make an explicit statement to diminish the possibility that the family's resistance is being exacerbated by guilt or feelings that they are being blamed by the therapist. For example, the therapist might say, "While we don't believe families cause problems like Phillip's, we do know that children with problems like his get better much faster if the whole family gets involved in finding a solution."

By emphasizing the need for the family's involvement as a way of helping to cause change, the message that they are to blame is neutralized, and the family's anxiety may be decreased sufficiently to allow therapy to begin. Such a message may be particularly useful when working with families of chronic patients who may have had many negative experiences with mental health systems that, in fact, have blamed them implicitly or even explicitly.

Problem 2. The resistance is defined as located in another family member

Often, the family member making the phone call defines the resistance as located in some other part of the system, some part with which the therapist is not in contact. The most common unavailable or resistant member, especially if one works in a child guidance clinic, seems to be the father. The wife/mother is usually left to explain. The phrase "I would be happy to come, but my husband can't/won't come" epitomizes the message she carries to the therapist.

For example, Mrs. Carter brought her 16-year-old daughter, Mary Jane, to the emergency room following a suicide gesture. A few questions about the family situation included as part of a larger screening interview revealed a great deal of family conflict, and a decided rift in the marital relationship, with Mrs. Carter overtly siding with her daughter against her husband. Mrs. Carter's response to the recommendation of family therapy was to list the reasons why her husband couldn't and wouldn't come. These ranged from the claim that he couldn't take time off work since it would jeopardize his job in "these hard times," to the assertion that he didn't really care about either his wife or daughter. She stated, "He works long hours. He doesn't believe in therapy anyway. It certainly would help if he could be more involved, but he just won't. We've tried for years."

SUGGESTIONS

Use the Family System to Involve the Resister. The therapist can accept the statement of the family member about the "resister" at face value, yet continue to investigate the family situation in an attempt to discover factors that could either provide leverage to get the refuser to cooperate, or factors which might motivate other family members to get them to come.

With the Carter family, this exploration revealed that Mrs. Carter had been in a chronic one-down position, and had tried to get her husband involved in family therapy in the same way she tried to get him involved with her, by nagging and wheedling. When the therapist asked how she had attempted to gain her husband's participation in past therapies, it became clear that she had repeatedly sent the message "Come with us to see the experts so they can tell you what I've known all along, that you are an unreasonable, uncaring bastard." Without knowing it, Mrs. Carter had been unwittingly encouraging her husband's resistance by blaming him for all of the family's problems.

Discovering a pattern in which one family member is actually encouraging the resistance of another makes it possible for the therapist to suggest different strategies for involving the "resister." In our example, Mrs. Carter was persuaded of the importance of sending a clear message to her husband that neither she nor the therapist were interested in blaming him or anyone else, but that problems such as their daughter's suicide attempt were serious enough to require the involvement of all family members, at least in the early stages of therapy. This message served the double function of overcoming the husband's initial resistance while beginning to change the unsuccessful way in which this woman sought to involve her husband with herself and her daughter.

It is often useful to convince the family member with whom the therapist is in contact that the involvement of the alleged resistant member is indeed crucial to the outcome of therapy, particularly in those cases where the lack of involvement of that member is encouraged by other family members. The therapist can stress the potential usefulness of "uninvolved" family members as resources in solving problems. For example, the therapist can stress the importance of a parent as head of the househld, of older siblings as important role models for younger siblings, and of mothers *and* fathers as the cornerstones of family life. In this case, Mr. Carter, a successful businessman, was eventually asked to bring his considerable executive expertise to bear on the management of his family.

The therapist may also appeal to the family representative to use other members of the system to deal with the resistance located in one person. In the Carter family, for example, the therapist, in addition to modifying the message Mrs. Carter gave her husband about therapy, asked, "Who in the family has the most influence over your husband?" Mrs. Carter said she guessed her oldest son, John, probably had the most influence. The therapist suggested she ask her son to help persuade her husband to cooperate. The oldest son was able to help his mother to persuade his father to participate "at least once." The phrase "at least once" is useful because most people feel they are not making a commitment or giving up much control if they agree to only one session. This gives the therapist a chance to make that one session helpful enough to gain ongoing involvement.

Challenge a Family Member. Variations on the theme of "You could get him to come if you really tried," are sometimes helpful. The therapist can challenge a family member to get the resistant member to come. This technique makes use of the positive side of the caller's ambivalence about having the resister come, and plays to their sense of competence and competition. This technique works particularly well with members who sometimes act and feel helpless but who have a strong side. It is also a good technique to use with parents who do not wish to admit, even to themselves, that they are so ineffective that they cannot get their own son(s) or daughter(s) to come.

During this process the therapist must be careful not to be co-opted into a premature coalition with the family representative who is locating the resistance elsewhere, except as a strategy to obtain the cooperation of other members. The therapist must help the caller to find ways of involving resistant members, without buying or reinforcing the view that it is only those others who are resistant. In fact, care should be taken to avoid reinforcing the resistance of other members by perpetuating the perception of either the cooperative or resistant members that the therapist is in a coalition with any portion of the family against another.

Call the Resistant Member Directly. The therapist may call the resistant member directly. This is particularly effective if the therapist suspects that the original family representative is consciously or unconsciously colluding in the resistance, but isn't giving the therapist much leverage to work with the collusion directly. This technique avoids one of the pitfalls of the go-between process, that is, the inevitable distortions of the therapist's message during its reinterpretation to the rest of the family. The therapist may find the reportedly resistant family member quite agreeable when the need for his/her participation is presented in a nonthreatening way by a source outside the family. The resistant member may simply want a chance to express his/her ambivalence, or may be in a power struggle with the original family representative.

There are potential dangers to this intervention, however, and it must be used carefully and diplomatically. Therapists must be careful to avoid the unspoken or unwitting communication that they are more competent than the caller who has failed at the task of getting the cooperation of other family members. This message will only enhance resistance on the part of the individual who was initially at least superficially cooperative. The therapist also must guard against taking too much responsibility for the work of the family. It is generally preferable to place the task of involving family members on other family members. In this way, therapy begins before the first session, as the family's own sense of relatedness, power, and ability to deal effectively with one another is reaffirmed.

Be Flexible in Scheduling Initial Appointments. It is a good principle to start out being as flexible as possible with resistant families or resistant family members. The therapist can enhance the likelihood of the cooperation of a resistant member by being especially solicitous about his/her convenience. The therapist may wish to reassure family members that appointments can be scheduled at times when they will not have to take off time from work or endure undue hardship. Offering an evening appointment, even if it means the therapist must work an extra evening for that particular week, may give the therapist the needed inroad with the family which will allow them to schedule earlier appointments on an ongoing basis.

When a therapist genuinely cannot accommodate to the family's convenience, it often helps to give a brief explanation. This communicates that the therapist cares about their request even when it cannot be accommodated. For instance, a therapist might say, "I'm booked solid that night except at 6:00 P.M. and I really would like to see you this week. Can you try to make it then, and we'll see about a better time for the future?" Obviously, reality dictates some limits to therapist flexibility, and therapists should not allow themselves to be bullied into masochistic schedules by resistant families. An emphasis on flexibility does not mean a therapist should wait patiently until 8:00 P.M. because a family wants to have a leisurely dinner before coming in. An appeal to a family's sense of fair play can be made, as in "Unfortunately, I can't eat until after our appointment so how about grabbing a snack to ward off starvation and coming at six?"

Problem 3. Specific requests to exclude some family members

Most family therapists assume that all family members potentially have a role in the maintenance of the symptomatology of a dysfunctional member, and thus believe it is important to get even "uninvolved" family members in at least for an assessment. Many families do not share this view. Troubled individuals may assume that other members of the family do not know about their problem, don't care about their problem, should not be exposed to it, or are simply irrelevant. For example, when a young woman with anorexia nervosa called to request treatment, she was quite willing to involve her parents but expressed great reluctance to involve any other family members. Although she was steadily losing weight and had been looking quite depressed for some time, she was convinced that her siblings did not and should not know about her problem.

SUGGESTIONS

Find Out Why. The therapist can begin by investigating the reasons the caller wishes to exclude certain family members. Often there is an overtly stated reason for wanting to exclude a member, such as the perception that he/she is unaware of the problem, too sensitive, or not interested. If the reason given for excluding a family member is their lack of awareness of the problem, the therapist can point out the reality, namely, that the other family member probably has not only noticed the problem but is probably quite concerned about it. Often people fail to realize how much others notice about them, assuming that someone has not noticed because he/she has not commented on the issue. Usually that person has not commented on the problem because of a wish not to intrude or add further upset to the distressed family member.

The young woman with anorexia assumed that neither her older sister who lived nearby with her husband nor her younger brothers who lived with her had noticed her weight loss and depressed affect. During the initial interview she was pleased and surprised to hear that they had not only noticed but that they were quite worried about her and frequently talked about it with each other. She left the interview with an increased feeling of having the support of her entire family in coping with her problem, even though she still did not believe it was necessary to include all her family members in ongoing therapy.

Offer Reassurance. Sometimes a major reason for excluding family members is fear that certain family secrets will be revealed. Frequently, the so-called secrets turn out to have been long known but not discussed. Mr. and Mrs. Taylor called to request therapy for their 16-year-old daughter, Susan. They were deeply concerned about her promiscuity. Although both parents were willing to come, they vehemently refused to bring Susan's younger siblings, feeling that they should be protected from the knowledge of their sister's behavior, that they could not possibly offer any help, and might, in fact, be permanently damaged by discussions of this nature. Since Susan's siblings were close to her age, attended the same school, and shared some of the same friends, this attempt to protect them seemed unrealistic.

It is possible in such cases to directly confront the belief that the problem is a secret or to reassure family members that the "secret" will not be revealed if they will allow the members in question to attend. In this case, the therapist promised not to reveal Susan's behavior unless and until it was agreeable to everyone. During the initial session Susan's 12-year-old sister revealed that she not only knew about Susan's behavior, but had been teased about it in school. She had been afraid to discuss the issue with her parents and therefore had been suffering on her own. The Taylors quickly realized that keeping this secret was causing, not avoiding, pain in Susan's younger siblings.

Similar approaches may be used to involve a family member who is being excluded because others feel he/she is too sensitive. In the Malloy family, for example, Tom was convinced that his wife, Edith, would have a nervous breakdown if forced to deal directly with their only daughter's plan to move away from home to a distant part of the country. He wanted to bring his daughter into therapy so that the therapist would convince her not to move, and he most decidedly did not want to include his wife in the sessions. The therapist bypassed a discussion with Tom about the appropriate use of therapy, recognizing a classic family problem in dealing with emancipation issues, and instead concentrated on convincing Tom that she would control the session in such a way that his wife's tenuous emotional balance would not be threatened. It seemed likely that either Edith was colluding with her husband to prevent their daughter from emancipating or Tom was using his wife's alleged frailty to avoid losing his daughter. During the initial interview it became obvious that Edith's anxiety was as related to her fears about Tom's reactions to their daughter's leaving as it was to her own. Over time, the therapist was able to help the couple deal appropriately with the loss of their daughter and to reinvest the energy they had focused on their daughter into their own lives.

Problem 4. Overt rejection of family therapy

During the first phone call, families may make direct statements rejecting family therapy. These statements usually sound something like "Frankly, we asked for individual treatment for Linda because she's so unhappy," or "We really came in for medication for John's depression." These direct statements are difficult to handle, particularly if the therapist has sympathy for people who come to an agency or institution with some ideas about what they want, but who get something else. Even if family therapy makes more sense, such people feel manipulated or feel that their opinions have not been respected. Those without the financial resources or sufficient knowledge of health care delivery systems to purchase the care they want in the private marketplace are especially vulnerable to such tactics. Because the system in which therapists work often decrees the type of therapy which is done by whom to whom, family therapists may have limited freedom to respond to a request for another kind of treatment; even if they wanted to. On the other hand, family therapists may believe that family therapy is the treatment of choice despite the family's feelings to the contrary. Most family therapists have an emotional investment in the efficacy of family therapy for a wide variety of presenting complaints. It is sometimes difficult for therapists who feel caught between the family's wishes and their own sense of what would be best.

SUGGESTIONS

Don't Argue and Don't Be Defensive. A person who is already annoyed at not getting what he/she asked for does not need an argument.

This might seem obvious, but it is at this very point that many therapists lose families by allowing a defensive or annoyed tone to creep into their voices, which comes across clearly to the family member. Already overworked therapists or overextended students may be particularly vulnerable to responding with irritation or impatience to these blatant refusals. Therapists, particularly those new to the practice of family therapy, must remember that family therapy is an irrational idea to those who have not been introduced to its underlying theories or who have not yet had a chance to see its benefits demonstrated. Unfortunately, some students of family therapy fall into this category and may feel they are being pushed to defend something in which they themselves have little faith.

Be Sympathetic. Encourage the family representative to express as many objections as possible. The therapist can even elaborate on these objections, saying things like "I guess our request for you all to come doesn't make much sense to you," or "It may be that individual sessions will be necessary; let's discuss that at the session." This technique usually takes the edge off the anger behind whatever the family representative is saying and predisposes him/her to listen to what the therapist has to say.

Leave Everything Negotiable. If a family has a multitude of questions and concerns, it may be best to leave all decisions suspended until the first interview. If they ask for individual therapy or medication, the therapist can say that all such requests are negotiable and will be discussed at the first session.

It is important to remember that people usually request what they think will be best for them. If they request some sort of drug treatment it is usually because they have been led to expect that medication will be the fastest, most effective way to help their distress. If the therapist instead insists on family therapy, they may feel the therapist is withholding quick, effective medication in favor of what they fear will be a long drawn out course of talk therapy. Or, when both medication and famiy therapy are being recommended, they may see the drug as treating "the real problem" and the family therapy as superfluous. The therapist may reassure the family member that if he/she agrees with the request after having had a chance to meet with the family face to face, to get to know them and understand their point of view, he/she will do everything possible to facilitate the request. The important point is to postpone the decision about alternative treatments until family members have come in, thus giving the therapist an opportunity to use leverage to prove the potential usefulness of the modality, and giving the family a real basis for an informed decision.

Give Information. Many times families simply are not educated about the aims or the power of family therapy. Therefore, it may be important to do a bit of education about its benefits. For instance, if the family claims that the patient's problem is so serious he/she needs his/her own therapist, the therapist may partially agree, saying that the patient's problem is in fact so serious that the patient needs the whole family to help in the treatment. In working with families with seriously disturbed members, it is sometimes even useful to cite evidence that family therapy does help to insure compliance with other treatment regimes and to prevent rehospitalizations.

Problem 5. Challenges of the therapist's competence

Another whole set of resistances arising during the initial phone call and/or in the first session relate to challenges of the therapist's competence. A range of inquiries might indicate that this is an issue: "Have you seen other families like us?" (which really means "Do you have any experience at this?"); "Do you have children?" (which really means "Do you have any experience at anything?"); "Is it Dr. or Ms./Mr.?" (which really means "Do you even have training?"). These questions are so common, and cause family therapists so much trouble, that a separate chapter has been devoted to them. For solutions to these and similar challenges, see Chapter 4.

The first interview: Variations on the theme of negotiating the family boundary

The first interview is often the most interesting part of the therapeutic process. It begins the initiation of the family into an alliance with the therapist to achieve mutually agreed upon goals. All of the principles useful in handling the initial phone call apply; that is, the therapist must consider how the referral was made, how the family's representative responded to the first phone call, and go about connecting with family members by starting where they are.

In the first interview, the therapist has the complex job of exploring everyone's view of the problem and dealing with everyone's resistance while tracking family interactional patterns and persuading the family to accept and participate in therapy. This interview, however, offers many more opportunities than a phone call to deal with the family's resistance and to involve them in an ongoing relationship. Once a family is in the office, a therapist has room and time to maneuver, and a chance to convince the family that therapy may be helpful. Novices at family therapy should note that the goal is to connect with the family, *not* to solve all their problems in the first session. When beginners feel pressured to do the latter, they become overly anxious and thus stimulate rather than diminish family resistance.

Establishing a therapeutic alliance

Even when family members are in serious conflict they at least know what they can expect from each other. In the beginning, however, the therapist is perceived as a stranger. He/she is an unknown quantity, potentially helpful, potentially destructive. Since family members don't know what to expect from a therapist the therapist must prove himself/herself. Many theorists have described the notion of the family boundary, that elusive division between the "we" of the family and the "they" of the outside world. To negotiate the family's boundary, the therapist must demonstrate understanding and competence as he/she meets each resistance, so that family members begin to allow the therapist a special, if temporary place, in the family system, one which is endowed with power, authority, and trust. In Chapter 1, the relationship of therapists to families was likened to that of navigators to captains of ships. Therapists, as navigators, have special skills which make journeys possible; but families retain control of their ultimate destinations or the goals of their lives. In other words, the bond formed by the therapist with the family must leave the family feeling they are still in charge of their destiny but with a clear vision of the therapist as in charge of therapy and competent to help them. This process has been described by many authors using a variety of terms, perhaps most explicitly by Minuchin as "joining." The process of effective joining helps to avoid a great deal of what would otherwise be resistance.

Resistance as a property of the system

Families naturally resist admitting the therapist into a position of power and trust for all the reasons they resist change in general and therapeutically induced change in particular (see Chapter 1). In the initial interview, resistance represents the way in which the family protects itself from undue influence from outside its boundaries, from an invasion of the "we" by the "they."

Negotiating the family boundary requires that the therapist be able to integrate any individual's resistant behavior with a systems approach to organizing data. Resistance should be perceived by the therapist both as emanating from individual sources and as an expression of the family system. The overt source of the resistance may move from one member to another, may be a collusion between two or more members, but only rarely resides consistently in one member. No matter how it appears, resistant behaviors represent the entire system's resistance to change. Because an understanding of any resistance must be integrated into an understanding of its function within the system, the therapist must always be prepared to handle an individual expression of resistance while tracking the system's response to any changes that occur as they do so. When a father who has consistently represented the family resistance to change abruptly gives in and changes his attitude and behavior, it is not unusual to see a previously compliant mother respond by suddenly expressing doubts about the efficacy of therapy or the value of her husband's changed behavior. It is important that therapists expect such shifts in the locus of the resistance so that they do not become demoralized when they occur.

Frequently, beginning therapists get caught up in the resistance expressed by one or two members, spending the entire initial contact struggling to overcome it. More experienced therapists usually can use one part of the system to effectively handle the resistance in another part. For example, neglecting to focus on the entire system, one psychiatric resident got caught up with the expressed resistance of Ellen, a depressed 16-year-old girl who had a recent history of severe weight loss followed by weight gain to the point of pudginess. While her mother insisted they were coming at Ellen's own request, Ellen revealed that she did not want to come and that her father had promised her they would not have to return after the first interview. While the resident had expected resistance in an adolescent, he had not expected this resistance to be supported by her father. Unfortunately, he was paralyzed by the father's unexpected sabotage. Feeling undercut, he did not deal with the father, but engaged the daughter in a discussion about why she didn't want to come. Had he been more experienced, he might have been able to use this opportunity to explore family relationships. For example, he could have encouraged the mother to discuss with the father why he made such a promise without consulting her. That move would have avoided Ellen's overt resistance and allowed the parents to begin to discuss one of their very real problems, their parental relationship. Their marriage had been in trouble for years and currently they were unable to engage each other even to help their daughter.

Families differ greatly in the amount of resistance they offer to therapists establishing themselves in a position of authority and trust. Some families have very weak interpersonal and intergenerational boundaries as well as very weak family/nonfamily boundaries. In these cases, therapists must be careful that families do not become too dependent, leaving therapists responsible for the goals as well as the means of reaching those goals. Other families may have weak interpersonal and intergenerational boundaries, but strong family/nonfamily boundaries. An experienced therapist learns to use the amount of initial resistance a family offers as a source of information about the family's boundaries.

A CASE EXAMPLE

In the following example, the therapist carefully negotiates a rigidly guarded family boundary of a family with weak interpersonal and intergenerational boundaries, establishing herself in a position of authority and trust.

Jason was referred for family therapy by the inpatient service of a psychiatric hospital during his second hospitalization. Both hospitalizations had resulted from overdoses of aspirin. These could hardly be called suicide attempts, as Jason presented himself to the emergency room so promptly that the manufacturer's initials scarcely had time to dissolve off the pills. Nevertheless, he was sending some sort of distress signal, as well as aggravating a serious intestinal disorder. Jason was living with his parents, Sarah and Jon, despite his 23 years of age, college education, and considerable musical talent. While away at school, Jason had suffered a "nervous breakdown" during the final exams of his senior year. His parents rushed to the school, several hundred miles from their home, and stayed with him until he took his exams. Then they took him home where he had now been for a 3-year period without even trying to get a job or continue his schooling. During this time his main occupation had been to engage in screaming arguments with his parents, blaming them for his plight. His mother, Sarah, developed a severe depression which had been treated with antidepressants with no noticeable improvement.

Following receipt of the referral for family therapy, the therapist called the family to make an initial appointment. While Sarah answered the telephone, when she discovered who was calling she immediately said she would get her husband, Jon. Once on the phone Jon began telling the therapist the entire history of his son's problems. The therapist listened and commented on how difficult things must have been considering his son's serious problem. After being careful to hear the father out for a respectful amount of time, the therapist interrupted him to say that all this could be discussed at the first interview. Although the father persisted, the therapist continued to suggest that the initial interview was the appropriate place to discuss this information. The father stated that he could not discuss these issues adequately in his son's presence, and therefore, he could not have his son at the first interview. Since he would not back down from this position, the therapist agreed to a session with the parents alone, and an appointment time was arranged.

This phone call began the therapist's first negotiations of the family boundary. The therapist did not insist on talking with Sarah, but noted her behavior and planned to check out its meaning as the assessment continued. (Was this deference to her husband or a reluctance to get involved?) The therapist also set some benign limits with Jon in terms of his requests, in part to establish herself as in charge of the therapy, and also to establish a beginning rule of talking about the problem as a family, without separate dealings with the therapist. Following his acquiescence in saving his complaints about his son for the first interview, she avoided a power struggle over Jason's presence which she saw she wasn't going to win.

Immediately following the introductions at the beginning of the initial interview, the father pulled out a "psychiatric history" he had compiled going back to Jason's days at a child guidance clinic when he was 9 years old. He insisted on reading his list of dates and complaints, most of which were already described in Jason's chart. The therapist allowed the father to complete his list, nodding respectfully at points which he emphasized. Then she asked his permission to speak to his wife, Sarah, about their son. He gave the therapist permission, despite the inpatient team's complaint that he never let her say a word. Sarah immediately began to talk about her own depression, linking her feelings with those of her son. She stated that when one of them was down, the other was down. Jon agreed and commented that at one point both mother and son had been hospitalized so that he had been running from one psychiatric hospital to another in order to visit them both.

The therapist had noted in the first phone call that the father regarded himself as responsible for maintaining the family boundary. Sarah's immediate response of handing over the phone to her husband and Jon's behavior in presenting Jason's psychiatric history were all signs that the only acceptable point of entry into this particular family was through the father. The therapist was, therefore, respectful of him and his role to the point that she asked his permission to speak to Sarah. It was only after he gave his permission that Sarah felt free to tell the therapist that she suffered from depression. Her comments linking her depression to her son's coupled with her husband's overcontrolling manner quickly revealed that while the boundary between the family and the outside was a rigid one, there was an appalling absence of interpersonal boundaries within the family.

In this case, the therapist was successful in negotiating the family boundary and allying herself with Jon, the person in the family most in a position to determine whether therapy would continue or whether the family would drop out. In many cases, resistances succeed in thwarting therapy because the therapist fails to connect with the family power structure and thus fails to negotiate the family boundary successfully. Fortunately, there are some general principles to follow which make it more likely that this process will succeed.

Make It as Easy as Possible to Get a Therapist. Most families seek therapists in one of two states, either in an acute crisis that is disrupting their lives or with chronic discomfort which has temporarily exceeded the family's stress tolerance level. The benefits of rapid response to families in crisis has been well documented. The benefits of speedy response to families with chronic discomfort, however, have been underappreciated. It must be emphasized, therefore, that the temporary intolerance that occurs during a crisis in a family with chronic dysfunction offers an opportunity to change long-standing and otherwise rigid patterns. In fact, if therapy is available when the family is in either type of crisis, the boundaries of the system are more easily negotiated. Distress or desperation make family members more open to the idea of external input and new ways of relating to each other. The therapist has the opportunity to prove his/her worth immediately, and thus gain an instant toehold in the system. Such a toehold gives the therapist a greater chance of being listened to on an ongoing basis. For these reasons, family therapy is easiest if an appointment can be scheduled within 24 hours of the first phone call. If an immediate appointment is not possible, an extended telephone contact should be made, during which the therapist begins to deal with the anxiety of family members. Frequently, anxious family members can be reassured simply by a person asking all the right questions and providing support and structure.

Start Where the Family Is. It is likely that the family will want to start with a discussion of what they perceive the problem to be. The way in which the therapist conducts this discussion is part of starting where the family is. If he/she is successful in adapting his/her style and technique to meet the family's needs the therapist will probably have gone a long way toward negotiating the family boundary. No one wants a navigator in Boston or Baltimore who only knows how to get out of New York. Yet, some therapists behave like just such a navigator. They ask a family to respond to their routines which they apply without regard to the needs of a particular family at a particular time. Therapists will be more successful if they can be flexible in adapting their methods to the family's needs. For example, some therapists rely on a detailed history in order to make their assessment and treatment plan. Should they insist on taking a history with a disorganized family which perceives itself as in crisis, rather than addressing the crisis first, they will usually lose the family altogether. Similarly, a family which employs an intellectual style and expects to give a history as the proper way of beginning therapy, as Jon insisted on giving Jason's history, will be put off if the therapist refuses to listen to historical data and only asks questions concerning the present.

The need for therapeutic flexibility also extends to therapist style, which should in part be based on the style of the family. The same therapist who was quiet and respectful in her approach to Jon and Sarah, might well find it advisable to be breezy and perhaps even a bit humorous with another family. Being flexible, however, does not mean that the therapist should be a chameleon concerning theory. Flexibility has more to do with adapting one's theoretical and practical position to the needs of a particular family at a particular point in time.

Do Something Immediately Helpful. It is not necessary to produce startling change in the first interview but it is important to do something which family members perceive as helpful. This may be as small as relabeling some behavior as "not so crazy," or their situation as "not so bad, I've seen worse," or simply helping them sort out and sum up what they see as problematic. Since many times people come to therapy without a very clear idea of what they want except the cessation of distress, another immediately helpful function the therapist can perform is that of helping the family to sort out their goals. Whatever the therapist chooses to do, the family must be left with a sense of increased hope and belief in the possibility of change.

Leave the Family in Control of Their Fate. Negotiating the family boundary and being admitted to a position with some authority does not mean taking over altogether. Families must leave the first contact with the therapist believing in their own resources and abilities, not dependent on the therapist. In part this is done by helping them to make their own decisions about what their goals will be.

The whole question of who sets goals in family therapy has been a knotty one because of the greater degree of responsibility for change that most family therapists accept, and their use of manipulation to produce change. It is not necessary or desirable that family members understand or agree with all of the therapist's implicit goals for the family, particularly such general ones as "less enmeshment." It is, however, quite necessary that the therapist understand and agree with the basic goals of the family, as goals unacceptable to the family are impossible to attain. For example, the therapist for Jason, Jon, and Sarah had some goals for the family which were never verbalized, but which were possible to attain because they facilitated the family's goal, namely, to get Jason to stop taking pills and do more productive things with his life. The family could not have cared less about the therapist's concepts of "differentiation," "personal boundaries," and "autonomy."

Once an agreement has been reached about the goals of therapy the therapist must be free to use any techniques he/she possesses to attain them. While any technique can be regarded as legitimate if used to attain the family's own desired ends, techniques which involve paradoxical injunctions seem to some therapists to be offensive or downright unethical. However, if such methods enable a family to move from an impasse that is painful and intractable, they are appropriate methods of intervention. As navigators, therapists know best how to guide ships, and ships fighting the currents may be more easily moved by going at angles to the wind rather than directly fighting the forces of nature. It is important to recognize, however, that strategic techniques require great skill and confidence on the part of the therapist. For this reason, if a therapist is made uneasy by the prospect of employing such interventions, he/she should refrain from using them.

To summarize, the principles involved in successfully negotiating the family boundary are similar to those involved in using resistance to achieve change at any stage in family therapy. They involve being available when the family perceives the need for help, being able to demonstrate competence in understanding what the family perceives to be their problem, while remaining flexible in choosing the therapeutic role, and leaving the family in charge of their own fate while guiding them toward the agreed upon goals.

The first interview: Common expressions of resistance

Problem 1. He's/she's the problem, or I'm the problem

Although this issue is presented in our discussion of the first phone call, it is again stressed here since it is the most common form of resistance in early family therapy and, therefore, often will arise also in the first interview. Family members will tend to have a clear idea about who is the problem and who is symptomatic. Even if the therapist can see that certain family issues contribute to the problem as the family sees it, it is inadvisable to discuss this observation in the first interview. A common mistake many family therapists make is to immediately try to change the family's point of view. For example, an inexperienced therapist might have pointed out to Jon and Sarah the implications of their tolerance of Jason's prolonged dependency, the implication being that they needed him to give their lives meaning and purpose. Presumably such an intervention is an attempt to assume a systems stance by making the family the patient and making the victim of the family's complaints more comfortable by spreading the blame around. Since many therapists tend to be rescuers by nature, this is an easy and dangerous pitfall. Maintaining a systems perspective does not mean telling everyone everything you think. No good individual therapist hits a patient over the head with his/her most powerful interpretation in the first few minutes of therapy, and there is no reason why a family therapist has to do it.

Another reason therapists redefine the family as the problem too quickly is that while the family is fixated on Johnny not behaving right, the therapist sees other problems that are screaming for attention. One of our younger staff recently asked for a consultation about a family whose problems overwhelmed her during the initial interview. The family consisted of a father with a hearing impairment, two beautiful teenage girls who had inherited his hearing impairment, a difficult foster son, and one harried mother. They had been coerced into treatment by the Child Welfare Department because they couldn't decide whether to adopt the 12-year-old foster son, Larry — and no wonder. This boy had a troubled history of being moved from home to home as a small child. Although he was obviously very bright, in fact quite a bit brighter than any of the members of the natural family, he was also very disturbed.

Our young staff member spent the first interview alternately feeling intimidated by Larry, who kept the focus on himself by threatening physical violence to the therapist and refusing to ever come again; feeling appalled at the low self-esteem of the beautiful but impaired daughters; and feeling overwhelmed by the helplessness of either parent to control Larry. She finally asked the father to take Larry out of the room when she couldn't stand the provocation any longer. Fortunately, she ran out of time before she was able to attempt to expand the family's focus to include what she saw as their other equally serious problems. While she was quite right that the family had other serious problems, the family wanted to deal with the issue of Larry. Some improvement in his behavior and some decision about his adoption were necessary before this family could spend their energies on anything else. A senior clinician spent a session with the young therapist and the family demonstrating how to avoid "leaping through Larry's loops" in order to help the parents to establish some control over their young charge and get the therapy going in the right direction.

Although it is a mistake to attempt to expand the family's focus too quickly, it usually is also a mistake for therapists to agree with a family that locates the problem in one member. Sometimes it would be easy to agree since even the person identified in this way may agree, obviously demonstrating great distress. For example, recently a father called for treatment. His son, David, had exposed himself to neighborhood children. Rather than being angry with his son, or focusing on his son's act as a call for help, he focused entirely on himself. He was overwhelmed with guilt, seeing his neglect of his family as the principal cause not only of this son's deviance, but of his older son's recent death in an alcohol-related automobile accident. He vehemently insisted he was the real problem in the family. While his remorse was real, it dominated the initial interview to the point of obscuring all other issues, including the problems of his remaining son. David had been having many problems even before his brother's death; his father's guilt over that loss had further isolated him and obscured his escalating difficulties.

Had the therapist been oversensitive to the father's pain, she might have allowed family sessions to focus on his feelings of guilt, loss, and helplessness. Because of David's very real and immediate problems, she chose instead to arrange an individual interview with his father as part of the assessment process. At this time, she sympathized with his grief, but suggested that it was not useful for his son to see him as helpless. The therapist did not challenge his belief that his neglect was responsible for the family's problems, only the way in which he was reacting to those feelings. She suggested that the father had to pull himself together to give his son the feeling that he was strong enough to take control. This may sound insensitive, but it was crucial that this father continue to be a father to his son, even in his grief. Once David's crisis had been mitigated, it was possible to deal with the unfinished mourning of the entire family.

SUGGESTIONS

Leave the Focus on the Identified Patient. In most cases, it is not useful to move the focus too quickly off the individual who is identified as the problem by the family. They need to know that their concerns are being taken seriously and that the limits of their tolerance for change will not be exceeded. The therapist must bear in mind that however a family is organized, it's organized to prevent its own dissolution. That organization needs to be respected at all times, but particularly while the therapist is establishing himself/herself as competent to guide the family through the stormy waters that are bound to follow even small changes in an anxious family.

A psychiatric intern recently experienced a family dropping out of therapy after the older siblings of a 16-year-old identified patient hinted at parental discord. Following this hint he moved the focus to the parents, requesting that they unite to present the daughter with consistent demands. The mother immediately mentioned that doing so would stir up marital issues. The intern neglected to reassure the couple that he was not interested in their marriage, at least not at this time, that they were obviously capable people who had already successfully raised three children, and he was sure they could deal with their marital issues when they chose to do so. Instead, skipping this vital step, he escalated his pressure on them to discuss the potential marital disagreements during the week before their second appointment. The mother called midweek to request individual therapy for her daughter, firmly refusing a second family interview. Anxiety over the future of the marriage once the last child had emancipated had been stirred up before the intern had established himself as competent to handle the family's presenting problem.

Beginning family therapists who have been watching videotapes of experienced family therapists often make the mistake of moving too fast because they have observed senior therapists doing so. Sometimes therapists with considerable experience or therapists with international reputations can establish their competence quite early, and negotiate the family boundary so gracefully that their skillful moves go unnoticed by the beginners watching the tapes. Like a good quarterback in professional football they can "read the defenses" of the opposing team and call the plays accordingly. What would look to most people to be an unorganized attack by a group of behemoths can be seen by a Joe Namath or a Terry Bradshaw as a carefully choreographed pattern which frequently repeats itself. While experienced quarterbacks can anticipate these patterns and plan their plays, the rest of us would simply get run over. Family therapists can avoid the experience of being run over by a family by moving at their own pace rather than that of an expert.

Challenge the Identified Patient. The technique of challenging the identified patient is particularly useful if the family's presenting problems are vague or not severely pathological. Complaints that father isn't home enough, doesn't care for the children, or some other complaint about behavior which is not obviously dangerous can be handled by challenging the identified patient to defend himself/herself or confirm his/her family's complaints. This is essentially an extension of the idea of keeping the focus on the identified patient, but it is one which allows for the emergence of differences between family members. The therapist turns to the identified patient and says something like "Are you really as bad as these folks say you are?" or "You've managed to get your wife and kids ganged up against you." This works well in terms of getting family members to talk to each other and can be followed with reminders such as "Listen, you better tell her, she's the one who's complaining."

Problem 2. Cancellations

Even if the initial phone call has been fielded well, some families cancel or fail to arrive for the initial appointment. Their anxiety may have diminished enough to leave them with insufficient motivation to come to therapy, or their anxiety about therapy may be so high they have chosen to live with the ongoing problem. If this decision to cancel is an unambivalent one, there isn't much a therapist can do. In such situations, it is permissible to behave like the Alice in Wonderland character who just throws up her hands and says, "What's the French for fiddle-dee-dee?" — in other words, give up. Some families, however, cancel or avoid the first session in such a way as to communicate that they are ambivalent about coming, leaving the therapist a bit of leverage with which to work.

SUGGESTIONS

Explore the Reasons for the Cancellation. The therapist should first try to determine if it is an unambivalent cancellation or no-show, or whether there is some room to renegotiate. Nancy, for instance, had called to request marital therapy and had been given an early evening appointment time. On the day of the appointment, she called to cancel with obvious disappointment in her voice. She explained that her husband, Dick, had just started a new job and had to work late. Since his schedule was so unpredictable, she suggested therapy be put off until things settled down. The therapist was sympathetic about how hard it was to make demands on already busy people, and then began to ask a few questions about how the new job was affecting the marital situation. Nancy quickly confessed that if anything it had gotten worse with the new job, and that she saw marital therapy as more important than ever. Clearly, she was not resistant to the idea of therapy.

Define Therapy as an Aid, Not as a Stress. In this case, the therapist expressed concern about the situation and suggested that although it looked like just one more stress to squeeze therapy into their already busy schedule, she felt the stress for both Nancy and Dick would probably be less once they had managed to begin to talk about things and make some basic decisions about their priorities. The therapist sympathized with how difficult it was, but pushed Nancy to let her husband know how important it was to her to do something about the marriage. Nancy was able to get her husband to arrange to come the following week.

Offer to Call the Unavailable Member Directly so That a Convenient Time Can Be Found. To test out the degree of ambivalence in the decision to cancel, the therapist can offer to talk directly to the members who seem to be causing the scheduling problem. If the issue is not a reality one, the more cooperative the therapist is, the more overt the resistance will become. If the family member making the call accepts the therapist's offer, either the scheduling problem is real or the resistance currently resides in the unavailable member. In that case, a direct contact allows the therapist a chance to handle that person's resistances directly.

Problem 3. There's no problem

At a certain famous vacation resort, the staff are fond of responding to every complaint by saying "No problem." No matter what problem is raised, whether about missing luggage or the missing toilet paper in the bathroom, their answer is "no problem." What they actually seem to mean, as vacationers soon find out, is "It's not our problem, it's your problem." There are certain families who present themselves for therapy who have the same approach. It's the therapist's problem to find a problem in this nice, happy, all-American family.

These families rarely refer themselves to treatment, usually being sent by schools, child-care centers, or pediatricians who become concerned about the children. In one case, a child psychiatrist referred a family after evaluating their 5-year-old son Johnny at his school's request. Johnny behaved erratically and lacked social skills. His parents, Carl and Helen, came to the first three interviews and quite obediently and cooperatively answered questions and smiled frequently. The therapist could find no area that they considered a problem, even though he suspected from outside reports that the father had trouble holding a job and the mother would not venture from her home unless accompanied by an adult relative for fear of anxiety attacks. Furthermore, their 2-year-old daughter was already showing signs of disturbance, but neither parent thought her behavior peculiar.

SUGGESTIONS

Be Supportive. On some level, families such as these know there is something different about them or about their children, but they are too threatened to admit it even to themselves. It is best to allow them plenty of time to get to know the therapist before pushing them to look at their peculiarities. The therapist can begin by being supportive directly and by helping the family to get more from the people available to them. With the family mentioned above, the therapist focused on reinvolving each parent's family of origin, with whom they had been feuding, so that a support system could be created and some healthy reality infused into their lives. Therapists, however, must be careful to check out the roles that are likely to be played by the "supports" they are attempting to reinvolve. The authors have, on occasion, discovered what might be called "folie à whole clan," a condition in which extended family members add stress and reinforce dysfunction rather than alleviate it. Sometimes there is a good reason why the family has withdrawn from certain people in their lives, "cut-offs" being the better part of valor.

Invent a Myth. Families who feel too threatened by any kind of label which implies deviance will sometimes accept therapy in the name of someone or something else. Myths such as "We're doing this to keep the school principal off our back," or "Child welfare workers believe anyone but the parents; they always blame us, but what are you going to do?" serve to give families a rationale for cooperating in therapy without explicitly having to admit that they have serious problems. The therapist need not, and should not, verbally agree that the school principal is crazy, or the child welfare worker is unfair. Such a stance would only backfire as the family would use it to buttress their arguments with such systems. The therapist can, however, use the family's feelings about other systems to motivate them to come to and work in family therapy by seeming to accept such myths as rational reasons for coming to therapy.

Problem 4. One member dominates

Therapists who are not yet comfortable with their own power and the need to control a session often have trouble with the family member who tends to dominate the session. Such family members not only describe everyone's faults or issues in detail, but often answer the questions put to others and seem insensitive to the therapist's interruptions or attempts to encourage more equal participation. One-member dominance not only decreases the possibility of accomplishing the work of the session, but if allowed to continue also decreases the therapist's credibility and ability to help.

For example, a psychiatric resident reported that he had seen a mother and daughter who showed up without the rest of the family whom they claimed flatly refused to get involved. The mother began to talk nonstop about how bad her daughter was. Since this was his very first family interview with any family the resident sat helplessly by while the mother talked for nearly an hour. He had been trained to ask questions and listen carefully in order to assess the data and make a diagnosis, and that is what he did. The mother, receiving no response to her initial complaints, escalated until she was literally screaming, as her daughter sat passively listening, making an occasional face as her mother talked. Overwhelmed, the resident finally asked the mother to leave the room so he could talk to her daughter. He learned that she was indeed behaving as the mother said, that is, staying away from home as much as possible. She was so overwhelmed by her mother's intrusiveness that she put her life in danger by staying overnight in parks and underneath bridges or sleeping in fraternity houses with anyone who asked her. Clearly bowled over, the resident ran for help from his supervisor immediately after the session. Unfortunately, by the next week, the mother had decided there was no possible support for her side from a therapist who would put her out in the hall, the daughter felt no one could control her mother who would "never change," and the case was lost.

This is a somewhat extreme example of what can happen when one family member is allowed to dominate the initial interview. Sometimes the person is merely nervous about being in a new situation, being unsure of what is expected of them. People who are merely anxious usually respond easily to minor limiting interventions while those who are genuinely intrusive and controlling often persist unless the therapist is firm. It is easy to dislike these people as they are often angrily blaming other family members, previous therapists, or forces beyond their control for their distress. Many a case has been lost by a therapist who is irritated into a premature confrontation or a desperate tactic, such as the resident who excluded the mother from the interview altogether.

A variation on the dominance theme occurs when family members control sessions by the use of extensive verbal skills and/or superficial charm. In this case, rather than being overwhelmed, therapists may be seduced into allowing one member to dominate because they are impressed with that person's obvious insight into the issues and his/her ability to comment on the family's metacommunications. Unwary therapists find that the appointed time has slipped by without their learning anything about the family except what the articulate member wants them to know. One of our students encountered a case where the sensitive and articulate member was a very bright 12-year-old girl. The therapist was quite taken with her, and her parents were so proud of her precocious grasp of adult matters that all three adults spent the entire hour listening to her and beaming their approval. The student was still beaming when she came for supervision, thinking she had a real treat for her supervisor, unaware that she had been so dazzled by a 12-year-old child that, rather than dealing with essential family dynamics, she had joined the family pathology.

Beginning therapists are particularly vulnerable to the distractions caused by these articulate members for two reasons. First, they often believe the charmer has better insight into the family's problems than they themselves do, and second, they're so grateful that someone is talking that they are loath to discourage the process for fear that silence will result.

SUGGESTIONS

Reward the Talker but Move On to Other Family Members. After enough time has passed that the talker feels the therapist has dealt with him/her respectfully, the therapist can thank the talker for his/her contribution but suggest that it is important to hear from other family members as well. After acknowledging either their distress and/or their insight, the therapist can firmly move on to ask questions of other members. Truly anxious or intrusive people will find it difficult to remain silent and may continue to interrupt. The therapist should politely stop them, promising to get back to them in a minute, but insisting the other family members be given a chance.

The reason for all this politeness when it is not a social occasion is that in the initial interview, the therapist is still outside the family boundary and must act accordingly. Politeness tends to insure therapists won't lose families if they need a little time to figure out where they are going and what they are going to do. It doesn't hurt to remember the advice of the Red Queen in Lewis Carroll's *Through the Looking Glass:* "Curtsy while you're thinking what to say. It saves time." Once the therapist becomes a part of the family, he/she can become more direct. Rather than throwing her out of the session, our resident with the overwhelming mother could have said, "Mrs. Jones, I can see that you're very upset. I'd like you to take a few minutes to pull yourself together while I talk to Jennifer. I need to hear her views as well." He would undoubtedly have had to repeat his request several times, but unless she was overtly psychotic, the mother would have eventually quieted down.

Accuse the Talker of Doing All the Work. The therapist may suggest that by doing the talking, the talker is letting all the other family members off the hook. This is essentially the old relabeling trick, in this case, relabeling dominance as overresponsibility, self-sacrificing but inappropriate in this context. This technique works particularly well with anxious people who are pouring out their own guilt, rather than angry people who are accusing everyone around them. The atmosphere of the interview can often be lightened by a therapist who says, "Hey, wait a minute, Joe. You're doing the work for everybody here. I'll bet they had something to do with all this, too" (see also Chapter 4).

Use Physical Proximity to Limit the Talker. With very anxious persons or with children and adults with poor impulse control, the therapist may ask the talker to move into a chair close to him/her and announce that he/she is going to "help the talker" by putting a hand on his/her arm each time he/she interrupts. This is another intervention which would have worked well for our overwhelmed resident. It is important, however, that these offers to help by limiting talkative members are not done with hostility. If a therapist feels he/she cannot give this message in a supportive and comfortable way, the technique should be avoided.

Problem 5. One member won't talk

While some family members talk too much, some talk too little, or not at all. One member simply refuses to participate, either out of antipathy for the whole idea of therapy or because of the role he/she plays in the family. The latter is often true when the family also contains an intrusive, talkative member, so that frequently both forms of resistance occur in the same interview operating in a complementary manner. This is illustrated by the case of DV, Rose, and their adolescent daughter, Emily. Rose was a real talker, completely dominating the first 10 minutes of the first interview. The therapist managed to quiet her down and address a few questions to DV who ducked them by pointing to Rose and suggesting that the therapist ask her. Rose, of course, was only too eager to supply the answers. The therapist then asked DV why he wouldn't say what was on his mind since she was sure he had an opinion. DV shrugged and stated that that's just the kind of person he was, with a finality that might have convinced a less tenacious therapist to move elsewhere.

The problem of a family member who refuses to talk because of antipathy to therapy is commonly demonstrated by adolescents. Since adolescents are often coerced into coming for therapy, they may arrive feeling unrespected, angry, and belligerent. They have no other effective way of resisting their parents or the therapist other than refusing to participate. In the family just described, Emily's way of resisting both Rose and the therapist was to sulk in her chair and refuse to answer questions. When the therapist persisted, Emily finally burst out with "I told them I didn't want to come, and they said I had to. Well, I don't have to like it."

SUGGESTIONS

Challenge the Person's Definition of His/Her Role. When a person defines himself/herself as "not a talker," the therapist can challenge that role by insisting that everyone has an opinion and that his/hers is just as important as anyone else's. An emphasis can be placed on how important it is to hear from the nonparticipant. Statements can be made such as "I really need to hear what everyone thinks of all this," or "It will help me to understand what's going on in this family if you tell me what you think." In the case of DV, the therapist persisted in asking DV what he thought until he finally said he thought the family problem was a case of "not enough rules and boundaries," adding several cogent examples. The therapist was surprised to hear this unsophisticated rural gentleman give such a sophisticated analysis of the problem. She was left reminding herself that human wisdom is not the exclusive domain of mental health professionals.

Solicit the Antipathy. Silently brooding adolescents or adults usually should not be ignored if the therapist has a choice, although this is always a temptation. Their nonverbal expressions of anger and belligerence are communications. They should be encouraged to make these statements openly. By encouraging the angry person and listening carefully to his/her point of view, the therapist demonstrates a willingness to listen and a courage in dealing with anger. In Emily's case, the therapist acknowledged that Emily didn't want to be there and went on to ask if she often found herself doing things she didn't want to do to please her parents. This immediately struck a sympathetic chord and Emily began to complain more directly. This eventually led to a discussion of how hard it is to do things you want to do when you think someone else's feelings might be hurt, a prime problem between Emily and her mother.

Give Permission to Be Silent. If a family member persists in refusing to speak despite the therapist expressing obvious interest in his/her point of view, it is best to avoid a power struggle over their nonparticipation. Rather than coaxing the reluctant member to participate, the therapist can give him/her explicit permission to be silent. In Emily's case, had she not responded to the therapist's inquiries, the therapist could have said, "Okay, Emily, it's okay if you don't want to be here and even if you don't want to talk. Maybe if you just listen while your parents and I talk, it will be helpful. If you change your mind, and want to join in let us know." Often this type of permission is enough to make the resister feel less coerced and more cooperative.

Take the Avenue of Least Resistance. Alan Leveton of the Family Therapy Institute of San Francisco has what he calls the Leveton rule about power struggles, which is "Avoid them or win them." Since a power struggle over getting an adolescent to talk is one most therapists could not win, a way to avoid a power struggle is to temporarily move on to less resistant family members. For example, if an adolescent is obviously angry but answers the therapist's first few questions with monosyllables, the therapist can simply start pursuing issues with those family members who are more motivated. Frequently, the adolescent will feel misrepresented and begin to participate by starting to correct the comments of other family members. In other cases, the adolescent may feel more comfortable and less coerced as the session continues, and therefore spontaneously begin to join in. As it becomes clear that the therapist listens, is fair, and is useful, less cooperative members begin to see the advantages in more active participation.

Ask the Nonparticipant Not to Interrupt. In this maneuver, the therapist challenges the silent member by asking him/her to be silent. As Milton Erickson has suggested, as long as people are going to resist you may as well ask them to do so (Haley, 1973). This technique puts the resister in the position of having to talk or give in to the therapist's order. It also tends to heat up the conflict, so it should be avoided if the therapist wants to reduce anxiety rather than escalate it. In general, remember, paradoxical techniques require unusual skill and the ability to quickly assess the function of any behavior in the system. Therefore, using such a technique in this ad hoc way should be done only with caution.

Focus on the Concrete. Sometimes nontalkers are resisting participation because the therapist has moved too quickly into threatening waters. In early therapy, this is particularly problematic since the therapist has not established trust or control and the family members may fear what they say will be used against them once they leave the therapist's office. If the therapist isn't a fan of samurai therapy, the quick and violent approach, it is best to focus on concrete issues and stay away from everybody's feelings. Anyone who's so angry he/she doesn't want to talk is hardly in the mood to discuss his/her feelings. If the talk is kept to safe subjects, such a person might join in.

Problem 6. The family insists the focus be on historical
     information

While this focus would not be a problem for a family therapist with an historical focus, the family that dwells on the past is a real thorn in the side of the therapist with a here and now view of the process of change. Some families cannot give up the idea that if only they can understand the past, they can fix the present. Given the long-term dominance of psychoanalytic thought in popular psychology and the dominance of linear causality in most reasoning processes, it is not surprising that many people tend to want to focus on historical information. However, if even one member feels this way and insists on dominating the initial sessions with his/her search for causality in the family's history, the therapist and the family can get bogged down in endless details. For example, a physician came to our clinic with his anxious wife and depressed 21-year-old daughter. He insisted on tracing the trouble back to when his daughter was 13, and obsessively went over details of her adolescence, when she had done this, when that girl friend had stopped seeing her, and so on. The therapist allowed this for a time and then slowly tried to move him to discuss more present and family oriented issues, but to no avail. His overt notion, especially understandable for a physician but common to many people, was that if he could find the cause, he could find the cure. His covert notion was also to establish the cause of his daughter's problems as extrafamilial.

SUGGESTIONS

Pose the Question of Relevance. When a focus on the past becomes unproductive or doesn't fit with a therapist's theoretical model for bringing about change, the therapist can politely raise the question "So what?" Families and individuals who obsess about historical details in the belief that if they find the cause, they can find the cure are hard to argue with since that's such a logical approach. However, if they are allowed to run with it, but with frequent interruptions from the therapist who asks the significance of their point as to the here and now, they usually eventually give in. In the case of the doctor and his depressed daughter, the therapist kept saying such things as "Okay, Dave, so Karen was 13 when her best girl friend started dating and stopped being interested in her. How's that going to help her now?"

Be Alert to Signs of Mourning. Before therapists employ the "So what?" technique, they should always be sure the obsessive focus on the past is not a sign of unresolved grief. Some people think they have reached some sort of resolution of their grief over a loss only to find that their feelings are still greatly affecting their current relationships. In these cases, a direct focus on the loss is usually necessary before the focus can be redirected to current problems. Signs of unfinished mourning usually appear as unusual affect attached to past events. Talking about the past usually lowers affect, so that if affect increases when historical material is mentioned, the therapist should be alerted and pursue these issues.

Problem 7. The family refuses to focus on historical information

Some families do not want to give any historical information at all because they are so caught up in their current experience that they regard talking about past events as a waste of time. This is particularly true of families in crisis and families with high levels of affect. They perceive the therapist as not understanding their level of distress when he/she wants to gather data about events in the past. However, historical information is vital to some models of family therapy or to a therapist's comprehension of a family's problems. Not all family problems are the result of recent issues or current stresses. Some problems are buried in a family's history, and are expressed in the present by family cut-offs and resentments which have been harbored for years without expression or resolution. A stubborn focus on the passions of the moment may mask the depth of these long-term unresolved feelings between family members.

Sometimes, historical information changes the therapist's perception of family issues or even redefines the problem. For instance, Larry and Donna presented for marital therapy due to increasing conflict. Donna complained that her husband was domineering and overly interested in sex. Larry complained that everything had been fine between them until Donna had attended a woman's group and had gotten all these new fangled ideas about women's liberation. In the first session, Donna admitted that she was more resistant to her husband's directives, but also claimed that he was more irritable and irrational. A history was taken, despite the fact that this battle looked like a classic example of the impact of current cultural changes on an old-fashioned marital contract. It was discovered that Larry's father and grandfather had died of Huntington's chorea. Since hypersexuality and increased irritability are early symptoms of this disease, a medical workup was suggested. While neither the couple nor the therapist had thought that history was likely to be important, it turned out that Larry did have this serious illness. This information was crucial to the focus and direction of therapy, and prevented an overemphasis on psychological interpretations of his behavior.

SUGGESTIONS

Provide a Rationale. Families in distress who balk at providing historical details need to be given a reason to put aside their current concerns. If the therapist can give a good reason for discussing these issues, family members will usually comply. Sometimes the rationale given may be that it is just good clinical practice to explore the family history for key events and previous physical or mental illnesses. Sometimes the rationale may be provided by the presence of three-generational patterns (see Chapter 5). Therapists can explain that while it seems pretty obvious to everyone what the problem is, they don't want to be careless in making assumptions, and past history may provide an added perspective on current problems.

Request Individual Sessions. When family members are so upset with each other that they cannot discuss historical matters without interrupting each other and beginning to quarrel, it is sometimes a good idea to see each family member individually to gain an understanding of their perceptions of the reality of the situation and how it evolved. This is particularly important in marital therapy when the presenting problem is explosive, such as the violent reactions of one spouse to the other having had an affair. It is also useful when parents and their adolescent children arrive at the first interview so angry that they cannot speak civilly to each other. Joining with each family member individually before bringing them all together gives the therapist a little added leverage and control, and gives the family a chance to simmer down.

Summary

Resistance is a normal phenomenon and is usually particularly apparent in the beginning of therapy. During the initial phases of treatment, it is sometimes difficult to distinguish between genuine resistance and family and systems realities that impede the family's commitment to therapy. Therefore, all behaviors should be evaluated in the context in which they occur. Factors affecting the level of resistance in any family include such factors as the health care system's response to the family, the way in which the referral for family therapy is made, the availability of therapy, past experience with other therapists, conflicting schedules of family members, differing levels of sophistication about psychotherapy, and class or cultural differences.

Resistance is a property of the whole family system. It may be persistently expressed by one member or it may move from member to member, but in either case, it always represents the resistance of the system to change. The guiding principle in handling early resistance is to avoid confronting resistance directly in order to get a foot in the door. At this stage, there is no strong bond between the therapist and the family which will help them to tolerate negative interactions, nor does the therapist know the family well enough to predict where and how resistance will erupt. The task of therapists is to persuade families to accept therapy by demonstrating in the phone call and the first interview that they are competent, understand each family member's experience within the family, and can do something useful to help them with their problems.

3. Contract-related resistances

ALICE: Would you tell me, please, which way I ought to
go from here?
THE CHESHIRE CAT: That depends a good deal on
where you want to get to.—Lewis Carroll

In family therapy, a treatment contract is an agreement between therapist
and family to work together on issues the family finds problematic in
order to reach specific, attainable, and mutual goals. While a contract is
an important part of the treatment process in any form of psychotherapy,
so little is written about treatment contracts in the family therapy literature that some might conclude that they are rarely a part of this treatment
approach.

Nevertheless all family therapists make either implicit or explicit contracts with the families they treat. All behaviors of the family and the therapist, whether or not they are labeled as part of the therapeutic procedure,
set precedents which become a part of a family's expectations of the therapist and of their notions of what will be expected of them. These precedents establish the rules and goals of therapy, and the roles that each person will play in the process of attaining them, thus defining the terms of
the contract. For example, a therapist who in the early stages of the first
session recognizes a deadlock between an adolescent and his father and in-
tervenes to arrange a negotiation of the issue is defining the role of the
therapist, the roles of family members, and what will happen in therapy
sessions.

Once family therapists are experienced, implicit contracts may work
well. Experienced therapists tend to know where they are going and what
must be done to get there. Experienced therapists also find it easier to keep
track of the metacommunications of their own and the family's behavior,
making it less likely that they will unwittingly establish precedents that are
not in the best interests of therapy.

For most family therapists, and particularly for beginners, an explicit
contract is preferable for a number of reasons. First, beginners are more
likely to have problems maintaining a consistent focus. In any given family session and in the overall process of therapy, they are much more likely
to become overloaded with information and to become temporarily dis-
tracted or permanently confused. Explicit treatment contracts avoid this

problem by providing an outline for treatment, helping therapists to organize the data presented by families, and enabling them to delineate problems and translate them into a realistic focus for treatment.

Second, beginners are much more likely to set inappropriate goals which are too limited or too ambitious, or which are just not consistent with those of the family. They may set goals which are not mutual; that is, they are their own goals or the goals of family members with whom they have been drawn into an alliance, rather than goals which encompass the needs of all family members. The very process of negotiating an explicit contract helps beginners to clarify the issues, the family members' priorities, and what goals are realistic given the nature of the problem and the resources of the family.

Third, beginners are more likely to be emotionally reactive to the behavior of family members, failing to evaluate the meaning of new issues in the light of overall goals. They may deal exclusively with a new and seemingly important issue when it really is only serving as a distraction from a topic that was beginning to get uncomfortable. For instance, when marital issues heat up a beginning therapist is more likely to allow parents to discuss the obnoxious behavior of their child. An explicit treatment contract provides a yardstick against which beginners can compare their own and family members' behavior to determine if they are working toward their goals or are off on a tangent.

Finally, explicit contracts help all therapists to set limits and establish control of the treatment process. By explicitly discussing and getting the family to agree about the goals and ground rules of treatment (such as who is to attend and what is to be discussed), therapists establish an automatic way of dealing with later resistances and challenges. If families want to drop out of treatment when the going gets rough, therapists can remind them that they agreed to 10 sessions. If a family member resists attending sessions, both the family and the therapist can point to that member's earlier commitment. Minimally, contracts enable therapists to spend less time policing the sessions and more time on the work of therapy. Maximally, the establishment and use of contracts can *be* the therapy.[1]

Therapists sometimes have trouble formulating good contracts for two reasons: They believe that negotiating an explicit contract means sharing their every observation and plan with family members, and they believe a mutual contract means that all family members must agree on the issues and all must want the same thing. Nothing could be further from the truth.

Being explicit about problem formation and the goals of therapy does not necessarily mean a therapist must be explicit about his/her own basic

---

1. See the work of Nathan Epstein and his colleagues on problem-centered systems therapy for one of the most effective examples of the use of explicit contracts.

assumptions or the means he/she intends to use to create change. In many cases, a discussion of these issues would provoke unnecessary resistance. For example, a therapist may observe that the parents of a teenage girl are much too intrusive into the details of her life, interrogating her each time she returns from a night out. Telling her parents that they are intrusive would only involve the therapist in a pointless power struggle. However, the therapist could formulate the problem in such a way that her parents could accept their becoming less intrusive as a means of reaching a greater goal. Such a goal might be their daughter's taking more responsibility for all aspects of her life, including bringing up her failing grades.

Creating explicit and mutual contract also does not mean family members must agree about every issue or subgoal. A family would not be requesting treatment if its members were in complete agreement. In family therapy, a contract may include different, and even apparently opposing goals for each member. For example, parents of rebellious teenagers may desire more obedience and compliance on the part of their offspring. The teenagers themselves may want more freedom to come and go as they please, and more privacy within the home. A therapist who wishes to make an explicit contract with such a family might encompass both goals in the contract by saying to the family, "I can see that you, as parents, need to retain some sense of control over your children to protect them from making dangerous mistakes, while you, as teenagers, need to start assuming some control over things which are important to you. I don't see these things as mutually exclusive. I suggest we meet together for eight sessions and at the end of that time we see if you are feeling better about the situation."

Either implicit or explicit contracts initially may contain radically different goals and/or rules for different family members. For example, if rebellious teenagers are unwilling to participate in therapy, they might be willing to accept a contract which initially only requires that they will come and listen. Their parents might be willing to establish a contract in which they will discuss the appropriateness of their rules, and their methods of enforcing these rules while their two teenage children observe.

It isn't only the therapist's level of experience that determines the degree of explicitness of the contract, but also his/her theoretical orientation. For instance, the contracts of behavioral family therapists are likely to be highly explicit, often including measurable goals, a specific number of sessions, and even written contractural agreements. Likewise, in Nathan Epstein's problem-solving family therapy (Epstein & Bishop, 1981), the contract is clearly spelled out and is a central focus of the process of therapy. Other approaches to family treatment, such as the experiential or psychodynamic ones, are more likely to leave these issues defined in more general terms.

No matter how much experience therapists have had, what theoretical position they espouse, or whether they eventually choose to use an implicit or explicit contract, it is important that they be aware of how their interactions with the family define the terms of the treatment contract. Since the treatment contract is so important, and since it is used to enforce the boundaries and rules of treatment, it is not surprising that it can become the focus of a great deal of resistance. This chapter will discuss how contracts are made and will divide resistances to treatment contracts into three categories: resistances to making a contract (contract formation), resistances to keeping a contract (contract implementation), and resistances to ending a contract (contract termination).

Contract formation: What's included in the treatment contract

Simply stated, the treatment contract spells out the boundaries of the therapeutic process. It defines the who, when, and where of treatment along with the goals and the overall means of reaching them. The simplest boundaries of treatment are those of the time, length, and frequency of sessions. Slightly more problematic is the issue of who will participate. The most difficult part of contract formation, however, is that of the therapist negotiating the family boundary while carrying on the process of problem definition and the setting of mutual, attainable goals.

Some therapists formulate contracts during the first session while others take several sessions to do so. Ironically, the simplest part of the contract negotiations, that of defining who, when, and where, often takes place after the more complicated processes of boundary negotiation, problem definition, and goal setting has already taken place. It makes no sense to deal with specifics before the family has had a chance to experience therapy and the therapist's style and skill.

The therapist's skill is particularly important in forming a contract because, as was stated earlier, families arrive for family therapy with each member hoping to change the behavior of one or more other family members in order to reestablish a disturbed status quo, that is, the way things were before someone rocked the boat. This is complicated by the fact that every family and every individual within a family, experiences a separate and special version of reality. Family members tend to see themselves as acted upon by the people around them, with their behavior being far more reasonable, given the situation, than that of other family members. A wife may complain that her husband is irritable and given to fits of temper, while he maintains that she constantly provokes him, subtly undermining his confidence in himself. A father may complain that his son is secretive and withholding, while the son sees his father as absent and unavailable.

Concretely, the first step in the contract process is for the therapist to get each member of the family to state his/her version of the problem, and then to spend some time investigating each person's response to and interpretation of what is troublesome. If family members have different versions of reality, it is the task of the therapist to translate all of these versions into a workable definition of the problem, and a viable agreement to change, with major goals on which all family members can agree. During this process, therapist establish their roles as experts and define the rules of therapy by the style and content of their methods of helping the family explore problems and possible solutions.

In contract formation, it is extremely important to start where the family is, never moving too quickly to a view of the problem that they cannot accept. The therapist must engage the family around what they have defined as the issue(s) that really matter to them. Lack of mutuality in this regard is a major cause of treatment dropouts. For instance, recently a new student saw a family in which the presenting problem was disagreement over rules between the youngest child, Carol, age 16, and her parents, Millie and Joe. It was obvious in the first session that Carol's two older siblings, ages 24 and 22, had not yet emancipated, and in fact were having difficulty separating from the parental home. In order to expand the focus beyond that of the identified patient, the student focused on this difficulty, making a metaphor about all three siblings needing to find ways of establishing rules for themselves in life without leaning on their parents. The parents, for their part, could begin to spend more time alone together. She left the interview with what she thought was an implicit but firm contract for the entire family to come to therapy to focus on this issue. She was amazed when only Millie, Joe, and Carol arrived at the next session and then only to announce they were withdrawing from family therapy and wanted individual therapy for their problem daughter. Belatedly, the student realized that she had moved too quickly to redefine the family's definition of their problem, and that she had unilaterally imposed what she believed to be the appropriate goal of therapy, a goal that was in fact quite threatening to them. She should have suspected that when a family's young adults have failed to emancipate there is usually a good reason. In this case, there was virtually no viable marital relationship between the parents. The potential loss of their children, a loss implicit in the therapist's statement of the problem, would leave them without the bond that held them together.

This student lost this family because she moved too quickly and too explicitly to explain her "systems" view of the problem. Although she was probably right in her assessment, it was neither necessary to share these thoughts with the family nor to move beyond their concern for their daughter at this very early stage of treatment. In such cases different goals must be negotiated at different times. Parents who are unwilling to focus on their intimate behavior or feelings for one another may well be willing to initially contract to change their behavior with one another *in order to help their children.* Later, if the children have become less symptomatic and the family has developed trust in the therapist, it may be possible to discuss the marital problems. The timing of the move to marital issues is all-important. After all, if they did not perceive the marital problem between them as being overwhelming, they would not have focused on their children as a way of avoiding their conflicts.

How treatment contracts happen

An example of a successfully negotiated implicit treatment contract may help to increase therapists' awareness of the way in which their interventions establish the terms and rules of this agreement. Let us return to the case of Sarah and Jon and their aspirin-swallowing son, Jason (see Chapter 2). As you might recall, the therapist carefully negotiated the family boundary by recognizing Jon's fierce protection of both his position in the family and the family boundary. Although she had a structural orientation and was not particularly interested in historical data, she listened with respect and initially did not challenge Jon's control of the interview. Only when he was finished with his summary of the problem did she make a move to broaden the discussion to include his wife. Taking a clue from the inpatient team's complaints that Jon never let Sarah say anything, she requested his permission to talk with Sarah before addressing her openly and directly. This left Jon in charge of the therapist's access to his wife. Sarah then broadened the potential focus of the treatment contract by adding her own depression and its connection with Jason's behavior to the list of family problems. Jon not only validated the legitimacy of his wife's problem, but also added himself to the problem list by spontaneously discussing the difficulties of visiting both his wife and son in their respective hospitals. Together these comments began to define the legitimacy of a focus beyond the identified patient. By this time, it had become obvious to the therapist that Jon was far too central in the family and Sarah far too overidentified with her son, both factors making it difficult for Jason to develop the competence and psychological boundaries necessary to enable emancipation to take place. Sarah and Jason seemed unable to express any opposition to Jon's overcontrolling behavior except as a passive, dysfunctional coalition. Since this mother–son coalition was disastrous to both of them, a more appropriate coalition was necessary. Jason could scarcely become competent at managing his own life while chained by his own dependency to his mother's depression and his father's control.

Since telling Jon and Sarah about these observations would simply have bewildered them and invited resistance around the definition of the problem, the therapist sought some other way to make the triangular nature of the problem a legitimate focus of the contract for family therapy. Following further discussion, Sarah admitted she had difficulty getting out of bed and frequently stayed there all day. The therapist commented on how difficult it must be for Jon to care for two dysfunctional family members. He acknowledged this difficulty, adding that he felt it necessary to keep everyone's medication with him at all times to prevent either his wife or his son from committing suicide. He claimed that he sometimes felt the family was a sinking ship. The therapist, seizing the metaphor, described the problem as one in which Jon repeatedly tried to keep the family ship afloat, while Jason tried to sink it and Sarah stood by helplessly. With Jon's permission, the therapist contracted for a change in Sarah's behavior, giving the rationale that she needed to help her husband to keep the family ship afloat, at least part of the time. The therapist contracted with Sarah for her to get out of bed every day by noon, get dressed, and cook both lunch and dinner for her husband. The initial interview ended at this point. Although a beginning contract had been established, it was by no means complete. Two members of the family had agreed on a family definition of the problem and one of them had agreed to change one current behavior, but as yet the third member had not been seen and the question of appropriate long-term goals had not been discussed.

At the next interview, after Jason had been introduced, the therapist carefully questioned Sarah about how well she had done on the tasks of getting out of bed, getting dressed, and cooking meals, even inquiring about her choice of menus. Sarah was quite proud that she had gotten out of bed and cooked regular meals during the four days between sessions, and her mood seemed slightly improved. The therapist's attention to the details of the contracted changes in behavior emphasized to the family the importance she attached to the contract. In all subsequent sessions, the subject of Sarah's cooking was at least mentioned, establishing and reinforcing Sarah's area of expertise and her contribution to the family.

During this session, Jason was presented with the modified definition of the family problem. Although he shrugged off the part of the metaphor about his trying to sink the ship, Jason was willing to go along with this new formulation. He and his parents were invited to negotiate appropriate goals for family therapy. The negotiations began with Jason's demanding custody of his own medication, and, with much intervention on the part of the therapist, moved to a discussion of what most 23-year-old men are busy doing. Eventually, three long-term goals were established which included Jason's finding a job or going to school, moving into his own apartment, and Sarah returning to her ice-skating lessons. She had begun taking lessons with Jon but had quit due to her depression. Jon was now quite good and performed with a group of senior citizen skaters. Sarah's return to skating would symbolize a move from her attachment to her son to take her place at her husband's side.

While the contract still emphasized Jason's dysfunctional behavior, the combination of a definition of their problem as involving them all and a list of attainable goals provided the basis for future therapy. All issues and events which followed were organized around this definition of the problem and this understanding of the goals. The therapist continued to encourage Sarah to help Jon by siding with him in disputes with Jason, or at least not interfering on Jason's behalf. Jon was slowly persuaded by both the therapist and Sarah to expect more from both Sarah and Jason, and to be less controlling and intrusive. Jason was the most resistant to change, and the last to show signs of improvement. He resisted taking responsibility for his own behavior, as he had when he had shrugged off the part of the definition of the family's problems which involved his behavior. The therapist kept insisting that he was responsible for his own behavior whether he liked it or not. For some time he continued to test the therapist by only partially complying with contracted behavior, and continued to antagonize the mental health system by periodically overdosing on aspirin.

After the second such overdose in a 3-week period, the inpatient unit recommended commitment to a state hospital. An emergency family session was held to discuss this recommendation. The therapist communicated the inpatient unit's decision to take a stand with Jason, repeating their view that if he insisted upon acting like a mental patient, he should be treated like a mental patient. Jon and Sarah implored the therapist to tell them what to do about this recommendation. The therapist insisted they make this decision together, an extension of her overall treatment strategy of encouraging Jon and Sarah to take stands with Jason, leaving the power in their hands. Jon and Sarah decided not to rescue Jason by signing him out of the hospital, thereby taking their first firm stand to limit his dysfunctional behavior. Jason, shocked by his parents' refusal, eventually negotiated his own reprieve by agreeing to go to a halfway house where one of the requirements was that he either hold a job or return to school. An arrangement was made with the halfway house to limit Jason's calls to his parents, and Jon and Sarah contracted to visit only once per week and not to contact Jason during the day when he was at school. Further, the importance of Sarah's continued participation in her ice-skating lessons was reiterated to prevent a reoccurrence of her overinvolvement with her son. Over time, substantial changes occurred. Jason continued to be abnormally dependent on his parents, particularly when making decisions, but he was able to complete his education and eventually got a job in another city.

By a continued focus on the treatment contract the therapist maintained the leverage necessary to engineer changes which forced a certain degree of separation and individuation in an enmeshed family. The original contract implied that the therapist would continue to work with the family as long as they kept working toward the goals. Some failure by family members to follow through on contracted behavior was tolerated by the therapist in an implicit message to the family that she understood the difficulty in changing patterns of behavior.

Common resistances to contract formation

The most common problems and resistances arising in the process of contract formation center on the unavailability of the entire family for family sessions, the unavailability of one member or key factions for treatment, differing views of problems and goals between family members, or between families and the therapist. Here, a few examples of each of these problems will be given, along with several suggested strategies of intervention.

Problem 1. Unavailability of family members, or "Joe works 3 to 11, father travels a lot, and I have classes three times a week."

Sometimes finding a time for the family and the therapist to meet seems to be an almost insurmountable problem. Although trouble at this early stage may be a symptom of resistance to treatment, it is important to recognize that not all families who have difficulty making regular appointments are resistant. The meaning of messages which communicate that the family cannot come must be evaluated for each family that presents for treatment. The context in which the message is sent is always significant. For example, one family in which the father worked out of town was only available for therapy on those weekends when he could afford the bus fare or could hitch a ride with his brother. In this case, the unavailability was not a measure of resistance, but a real-life difficulty around which the therapist had to work to get a contract. In another case, a young wife had difficulty scheduling regular sessions because her job selling real estate required very irregular hours, and those hours were at the convenience of her customers. The initial interview revealed that her job was a great source of support which balanced a marriage to a husband on whom she felt she could not depend. To ask this woman to risk losing her job so that she could attend marital therapy sessions which, in her view, might or might not have improved her troubled marriage, seemed antitherapeutic but necessary. It is unfortunate that, in order to begin therapy, family members must make their relationships a priority at a time when the family itself is least rewarding to its members, and when its very survival seems questionable. Nevertheless, difficult as such decisions and commitments may be, they are essential to the process of therapy.

The following suggestions constitute some good general policies for intervention, as well as some more specific interventions when resistance is the key issue.

Be Flexible in Scheduling Appointments. If family therapists are to treat other than the most flexible and motivated families they must be available during the hours most people are not working. Scheduling evening and weekend appointments can be a problem for therapists with families of their own, but it is important to make some evening and/or weekend time available. While professionals usually can exercise control over their work hours, factory workers and secretaries often cannot. Since some factory workers are on shifts which change frequently, it may also be necessary to change appointment times from week to week as the schedules of family members change. For most therapists, the discomfort of a schedule that is somewhat unpredictable is balanced by the satisfaction of more positive feedback from families.

Be Flexible in Who Attends Appointments. Unless therapists believe, like Carl Whitaker, that all members should attend every session or the session should not occur, they can be flexible about who attends sessions. For instance, they can work with those members of the family who can attend some of the time, but are not available for all sessions, as long as it makes sense in terms of the treatment plan. Planning who can make sessions must relate to the contracted definition of the problem and the goals of treatment. It is possible to have a treatment contract which is structured in such a way that the overall goals can be achieved without everyone attending every session. (Please note that this does not apply to cases in which members refuse to attend, which will be discussed later.) For example, the Family Therapy Clinic currently treats a dual-career family in which the mother and father are frequently out of town. The father travels to Europe every few months. His wife sometimes accompanies him, sometimes remains home, and sometimes leaves him in Pittsburgh while she travels on her own. Their severely disturbed 26-year-old daughter is the only family member always in residence. Her younger brother studies in Paris, returning for visits twice a year. The contract established with this family allows whoever is in town to attend sessions. The goals are flexible enough to allow for such an arrangement. When only the daughter is in town, she works individually with a psychiatric resident to diminish her obsessive anxiety. When her father is in town, family sessions focus on the problematic overindulgent father–daughter relationship. When her mother is in town, family sessions focus on diminishing hostility between the mother and the daughter. When both parents are in town, the focus is on the way in which they operate to unwittingly encourage their daughter's deviant behavior. On his infrequent visits, the younger brother participates in sessions to report the changes he notices, and to support his sister's moves toward autonomy.

Be Flexible in Spacing Appointments. It is not actually written in stone that appointments must occur at weekly intervals. In fact, Selvini Palazzoli and her associates (1978) believe that they achieve greater benefits by allowing a month's time between appointments, giving families time to react to and incorporate the messages from the previous session. In most models of family therapy, the estabishment and use of a transference relationship is not viewed as the major vehicle for achieving change, and therefore, the intensity and frequency of sessions required in traditional individual therapy is not necessary. Therapists may well find it advisable to try biweekly or monthly sessions, especially if weekly sessions are difficult for families.

Give the Family the Job of Finding Available Times. With very active and disorganized families, the therapist can become hopelessly bogged down trying to negotiate the question of time. Although many activities of family members can be modified or rescheduled much of the time, members of the family are the best judges of what should be given priority. By letting family members negotiate this task with one another at the end of the initial interview, the therapist not only gets an idea of each person's level of motivation but also learns something about the family's power structure and decision-making processes. If a family's priorities are a problem, the therapist soon knows it.

Make Home Visits. If resistance rather than reality is the issue, it is legitimate to bring the therapy to very resistant families, at least initially. Since people tend to feel more in control of their lives when on their own turf, an initial session in the family's home gives the therapist a chance to introduce himself/herself in a less threatening way. The therapist can demonstrate that he/she is capable of understanding the family's problems before the family has to deal with the physical reality of entering an agency or institution and becoming labeled as a "patient" or "client." Since the home visit with a very resistant family is an attempt to establish a link between the therapist and the family, a minimum amount of actual therapy need take place. A statement of some of the problems and an agreement by the family to come to the agency or institution is sufficient.

Problem 2. Omission of an important person

Sometimes contracts fail because the therapist has not included all the persons relevant to the problem at hand. Most therapists request that all family members come for an initial interview, unless the request is clearly for marital therapy. However, there are often key people who do not come or who are not a part of the immediate family, but who are intimately involved in the problem and without whose cooperation nothing will change.

Omissions of this sort are particularly common in single-parent families. A frequently omitted important person is the boy friend or girl friend of the custodial parent. While these persons often do not live with the family, they are usually an important part of what goes on. They may represent an additional support or competition for the time and emotional investment of the custodial parent. Along the same lines, the noncustodial parent is often left out of therapy sessions altogether even if he/she lives close by and sees the children regularly. The custodial parent is often hesitant to include the exspouse for fear of opening up the wounds between them, yet most separated and divorced people are no more able to cooperate with their spouses for the sake of children now that they are divorced than they were when they were together. The children remain caught between them in an ongoing, if somewhat more distant struggle. It's possible to involve exspouses in the same session, or to conduct parallel ones. Usually the explanation for the involvement of both partners is that they do not have to like one another, or even agree on most issues, in order to unite for the sake of the children.

SUGGESTIONS

Expand the Focus. Frequently problems which ought to be manageable but remain resistant to therapeutic change are related to persons and issues beyond the unit that is being seen. Marital issues may be related to the nuclear family, and those of the nuclear family to the extended family or the social network. Whatever the unit of therapy is, it often helps to expand it to the next higher level when therapy has reached an impasse.

For example, Tanya, a 12-year-old diabetic girl engaged in an incredible power struggle with her mother around administering her insulin, was referred to our clinic. She refused to inject herself and often would fight with her mother for more than an hour before she would allow her mother to give the injection. Although the nuclear family consisted only of Tanya and her mother, and both came to the first and all subsequent sessions, all efforts to support the mother's attempts to teach Tanya to take her insulin were to no avail, as her mother simply stated and restated her helplessness. As a way of discovering what was going wrong and who was important to whom, the therapist asked for a detailed description of their daily routine. Tanya's mother revealed that although Tanya's maternal grandmother lived over a mile away, she was a daily part of their lives. Every morning, Tanya stopped to visit her grandmother on her way to school. It became quite obvious to the therapist that in order to understand this mother's helplessness, she would have to meet Tanya's grandmother.

Invite the Missing Significant Person to a Session. Family therapy need not be limited to the nuclear family. In Tanya's case, the problem did not become clear until the therapist met together with the mother, the grandmother, and Tanya. While the mother and grandmother repeatedly denied any disagreement, the grandmother consistently sided with Tanya on all issues discussed in the sessions except the issue of Tanya's taking the insulin. On that subject, she merely shrugged her shoulders and looked as helpless as her daughter. The grandmother appeared to be unaware that her consistent support of Tanya on such issues as wearing makeup and tight jeans was rendering Tanya's mother incompetent in Tanya's eyes. Faced with opposition by her daughter and her mother, Tanya's mother had given up her attempts at setting limits with Tanya. It was only when the therapist persuaded the grandmother to join forces with the mother that there was movement toward the goal of Tanya's learning to inject herself with insulin.

In general, if a name pops up in a discussion or argument between family members, it is important to ask who the person is and how they figure in the family's situation. If they appear to be part of the patterns maintaining the problem, the therapist should ask the members of the family to invite them in. If the family objects on the grounds of not wanting to impose on these individuals, the therapist can point out that most people love to help if they are invited to do so. Therapists can reassure family members that most people don't directly offer help only because they don't want to be accused of butting in where they aren't wanted.

Offer Special Appointments. For family members who may fear being confronted or criticized, special separate appointments may be indicated. Exspouses, for instance, often fear the therapist, their exspouse, and perhaps even their children will gang up on them and use the session as a forum to criticize their behavior. One family practice resident solved the problem of the absent father/spouse by convincing the children that it would be a good idea if their father came in. He had first asked their mother to secure the father's presence, but she had claimed that since he didn't financially support them, he clearly did not care about them enough to attend therapy. The children were less caught up in their mother's resentment about the lack of support and thus were able to convince their father to come with them to a session held without the mother. In this way, the resident was able to establish two separate but related contracts, meeting alternately with the mother and children and with the father and children, both contracts geared to establish some consistency in the children's lives.

Older siblings living away from home sometimes are not willing to agree to attend family therapy regularly, particularly when it has been instigated by their parents because of the problems of their younger siblings.

Often they feel their own psychological separation from the family is so tenuous that it would be jeopardized by their attendance of family sessions. They fear emotional involvement with the family's problems through therapy will draw them back into the family system and destroy their hard-won independence. These semiemancipated siblings, however, are sometimes willing to make their own contract with the therapist. For instance, in one family where the youngest of three daughters suffered a short psychotic episode during her first attempt to leave home and attend college, the oldest daughter refused to attend family sessions. She was willing to come in by herself for an interview during which the family therapist made a contract to see her periodically. Since she was in daily phone contact with both her sister and her parents, she was able to use her sessions with the therapist to work out a more comfortable status with her parents as well as to encourage both her parents' and her sister's attempt to establish more appropriate interpersonal and generational boundaries. She supported the goals of therapy as long as the therapist did not force her to become reembroiled in the family cauldron.

Problem 3. Disagreement between family members about the problem

It is unrealistic to expect family members to have the same ideas about what the family's problems are, the desirable goals for family therapy, and who should have the major responsibility for change. A therapist who insists on absolute unity will fail. The task of the therapist is to find some common denominator in the needs and desires of all family members, or at least a common theme that will involve the family's most powerful and influential members.

A 36-year-old woman came for treatment at her husband's insistence. She had a 16-year history of an eating disorder and was currently existing on wine and coffee. She looked and acted very much like a Barbie doll, coming to sessions dressed in elaborate costumes and smiling inappropriately any time she made eye contact with the therapist. The negotiation of a working contract took quite a number of sessions, as it was some time before the therapist could believe the woman was saying what she really thought instead of what she thought the therapist wanted to hear. Her husband's definition of the problem was simple: His wife wouldn't eat. When her definition of the problem finally became clear, it came as a complete surprise to him. She claimed she had resented his controlling manner ever since they had been married. While she had obeyed him, smiling sweetly all the time, she had nursed a growing resentment of what she called his "Latin American *macho* attitude." To confound the problem, his mother, who lived with them on and off, was described by the wife as being as domineering as her son.

SUGGESTIONS

Find a New Definition of the Problem to Which All Family Members Agree. It is often possible to reframe the situation into a problem to which all sides can agree. In the case just discussed, the husband, while surprised, was willing to consider himself a part of the problem. It seemed reasonable to him that his domineering manner left his wife with little control besides her own food intake. Both members of the couple agreed that a more equitable balance of power was in order. She agreed to try to be more assertive, while he agreed to try to be less directive.

In another example, a young woman named Karen was well on her way to becoming a professional mental patient. She had been hospitalized 16 times between the ages of 17 and 26. She had had numerous diagnoses, ranging from manic depressive psychosis to borderline to schizophrenia. She had never seemed to respond favorably to medication, but it was impossible to measure its impact as she was whimsical in her approach to taking it. Karen's pattern, when psychotic, was to take off on "episodes" during which she traveled across the country looking for an imaginary lover. These trips endangered her life since she was careless about personal safety, sometimes hitch-hiking indiscriminately. Her father had to retrieve her from various cities across the country and bring her back to be hospitalized in Pennsylvania where she would quickly reconstitute. Upon release from the hospital, the cycle would begin all over again. She was seen with her parents who were understandably overinvolved with their disturbed and disturbing daughter.

During the first interview, Karen accused her parents of being intrusive. In order to establish some independence from her parents, she had moved from the suburbs to the city, taking an apartment a few blocks from the hospital. She found their anxiety about this arrangement to be intrusive. Her parents were defensive about their need to protect her, claiming to be in agreement with Karen's long-term goals but also claiming that she could not currently manage on her own. The struggle was presented to the therapist for resolution. Who was right? The therapist incorporated both Karen's statement of her parents' intrusiveness and their defense of its necessity into a statement of the problem. To Karen's parents, she said, "Considering what you have been through, it is understandable that you have trouble controlling your anxiety enough to allow her some space. However, if Karen is to assume more responsibility for her life, you have to give up some of it. Karen, you will have to begin to demonstrate some responsibility and independence in the shadow of your parents' anxiety. They will be anxious until you have proven you can manage your life a little better." Assured that they were not being blamed for their intrusiveness and that the therapist was taking their worries seriously, Karen's parents were willing to negotiate a contract which focused on a gradual decrease on their monitoring of Karen's behavior, a gradual lessening of monetary and emotional support, and a gradual increase in autonomy for Karen.

Make the Disagreement Part of the Problem. It is not necessary for all family members to agree on the definition of the problem. It's possible to say, "It's clear the two of you disagree about what's important. Let's spend some time discussing how you disagree, and come up with some ways of resolving this disagreement. We'll start with a discussion between you of. . . . " This technique is often useful when doing marital therapy when neither member of the couple is symptomatic and they have disparate versions of the problem. In many cases, discussion of the problem dissolves quickly into mutual accusations unless the therapist takes charge. Once the therapist has labeled the disagreement about the problem as an issue, he/she can begin to work with the couple on problem-solving skills and alternative ways of communicating with each other.

Ask Them to Give Up the Notion of Truth and Reality. An old story describes a rabbi who listens to a wife complain about her husband and responds, nodding sagely, "You're right, you're absolutely right." When the husband complains about his wife, the rabbi gives the same response. When the rabbi's own wife confronts him with his duplicity in dealing with the couple, he again says, "You're right, you're absolutely right." In fact, the *rabbi* is absolutely right. His response recognizes that each individual is right about the way *they* experience the situation. Since everyone perceives and experiences life differently, the notion of any one reality is not a useful one. Families must learn to understand what good therapists know, that being right is virtually useless in intimate relationships. No one can define anyone else's reality. What is important is how each person *perceives* the situation and how they feel about themselves, their family members, and their relationships as a result. The therapist can help couples to move from the impossible task of deciding who is right or what are the facts, to an appreciation of and respect for one another's version of reality. It doesn't matter if a macho man is really dominating, as much as it matters that his wife perceives him to be so. It doesn't matter if a wife really loves her husband, as much as it matters that he doesn't feel loved. These are the real issues for the treatment contract.

Declare Feelings Legitimate. A related strategy of intervention involves defining feelings as a legitimate part of the contract. When members disagree about the problem, it is often because one member is operating on the facts, while the other is focusing on feelings. Some family members refuse to see feelings as a legitimate part of reality. The therapist can help by explaining that, in therapy and in family life, feelings are important facts.

Problem 4. Disagreement between family members about goals

Even if people agree on the problem, they may not agree on the goals. For example, the Cooper family presented complaining that their son, Donald, was coming in late with beer on his breath, not cooperating in doing chores, and generally being unpleasant. Donald voiced resentment about the strictness of their rules. He and his parents disagreed over the goal of family therapy. They wanted to have more control over his behaviors, while he wanted them to have less. Disagreement about goals is even more common when couples come for marital therapy. Almost all couples agree that they desire "better communication" or "less conflict" but·these goals are so general as to be meaningless. What each person means by "better communication" and how it is to be achieved is another matter altogether. A wife may really want more intimacy while her husband wants more distance. In addition to the interventions suggested for dealing with differences in perceptions of the problem (all of which apply to goals as well), the following techniques may be useful.

SUGGESTIONS

Push for Specificity. Sometimes families have been engaged in struggles that have gone on so long that they proceed on automatic pilot, with polarized factions using "buzz words," anticipating one another's responses, and assuming they know how others think and feel. The real issues are obscured by mannerisms which serve to protect the members from the hurtful feelings of unmet needs and forgotten dreams. A serious push for specificity by the therapist often reveals that each person's real goals are far less objectionable than those everyone assumes to be in operation. Therefore, therapists must check out in specific terms both what people want and what they would be willing to settle for.

Label the Disagreement as Normal. In cases where the disagreement about goals is between generations, such as in the Cooper family in which the parents wanted more control and their son wanted them to have less, the therapist declares the situation absolutely normal and congratulates the family on their normality. This usually lessens the parents' anxiety over what they see as deviant and dangerous behavior and reduces the natural defensiveness of the offending adolescent. Resolution of the disagreement about goals then becomes part of the agenda for family sessions.

Use a Modality Other than Family Treatment. Sometimes the goals of family members are so disparate that it is impossible to obtain a workable contract to which the family can commit themselves, even when the therapist generalizes concerns. The most common version of this problem arises when one member of the family is concerned about other members who are totally lacking in motivation. Therapists should not be ashamed to admit that treatment of the family as a goup cannot work in every circumstance. When only one family member is motivated, it is possible to work with one member using a family perspective (à la Bowen) or to refer the individual to another treatment modality. For example, a family with an alcohol-abusing daughter came to the Family Therapy Clinic. The daughter claimed to want to control her drinking, and on the surface her family was supportive of this goal. In fact, they volunteered to bring in a severely handicapped sibling so that the therapist could accurately evaluate the stress in their home. Despite all this surface cooperation, the initial interview revealed a rigid and resistant family system with all members denying any stress other than the daughter's drinking, which they had partially resolved immediately by removing all alcoholic beverages from the home. Despite the family's denial of stress, the anxiety level in the room was extremely high, indicating tremendous tension between family members. In order to gain some understanding of these tensions, the therapist interviewed various family factions, beginning with the identified patient. This young woman indicated that she was quite concerned about the marital relationship between her mother and father. In a joint interview with her mother, she revealed that her mother would frequently drink too much and start acrimonious fights with her father. Her mother admitted to an intense hatred of her husband and stated that she considered her vindictiveness warranted. Although she was not particularly concerned about the relationship, she claimed that she was willing to consider marital therapy if he was. She denied any concern over her own drinking and stated she didn't mind the absence of alcohol in the house. When her husband was interviewed, he admitted to the enmity between him and his wife, but stated that he was resigned to the situation. He was devoted to his handicapped daughter and wanted to maintain a home for her. He regarded his wife's care of his daughter as excellent and was willing to put up with her vindictiveness in return for this care. There was simply no viable desire for change that could be extracted from this situation. The older daughter's request for family therapy had been a covert attempt to get help for her parents who sometimes figuratively tore each other apart. Her request to remove alcoholic beverages from the home seemed more related to her mother's drinking than her own. Once it became obvious that her parents were not willing to seek a change in their relationship, the daughter gave up her efforts to change them and agreed to therapy for herself.

Problem 5. Trying to form a contract when separation is
        a hidden agenda

Most family therapists are in the business because they believe in the institution of the family, and because they want to help people to make their relationships work. Sometimes this desire to help leads them to deny the fact that some couples or members of families come to treatment as a way of leaving a relationship. Fears of precipitating a breakup may cause therapists to make a contract to work on improving existing relationships despite blatant signals that an adolescent must be helped to leave home or a couple has come for the benediction "Go in peace. You're tried everything (therapy being everything) and it hasn't worked."

When the problem is a marital one, sometimes both partners want to end the relationship, but more often there is one partner who is more invested in maintaining the relationship than the other. When the less invested partner has already decided to end the marriage, there is no genuine wish to change and it is impossible to make an effective contract to work on the relationship. The disparity in goals is often apparent when, despite the efforts of one partner, the other continues to be hopeless about change even as change has occurred. Sally and Stephen presented with marital problems which had been worsening over a 10-year period. For the past 3 years their sex life, which had never been good, had become nonexistent. While Sally began by angrily listing a multitude of Stephen's sins, she relatively quickly moved to expressing how much she felt she was to blame, how much she missed the intimacy they once had, and how much she wanted the marriage to work. Stephen, who had laid the blame on Sally's doorstep, showed no emotion when she visibly softened and reached out to him. He continued to say that she would never admit to her role in their problems, despite her repeated admissions of this very fact. He reluctantly agreed to a six-session contract "to see if there was any hope." It wasn't until several weeks went by that the therapist and Sally discovered that Stephen was intensely involved in an extramarital affair. Even then Sally begged him to stay, but he insisted on a divorce. The signals in this case were clear, but the therapist chose to ignore them because she, too, wanted the marriage to work. Had she not been overinvested in saving the marriage, an alternative contract could have been offered that would have helped this couple to separate with dignity.

SUGGESTIONS

Help Family Members to Sort Out What They Want. Many people are not even conscious that they want to end their marriage or that they have already made a decision. When people have once cared deeply for one another, it is not easy to admit that the relationship is over or that one might have made a poor choice of mate. In the case of George and Debbie, both claimed they wanted to stay in the marriage, but needed some help in renegotiating their marital contract. They had been married in the Peace Corps in South America and had returned to the United States to finish their education. They prided themselves on their liberal marital contract in which extramarital sexual relationships were considered legitimate. However, Debbie complained that George seemed to be spending most of his time with the new friends he had found at school and that he had become involved in a dozen business projects, most of them highly specu-lative. George had no specific complaints about Debbie, although when pressed, he stated that he wished she was not afraid to ride on his motor-cycle. George was very fond of taking long trips on his motorcycle which he drove very fast. Debbie trailed along behind him in the safety of her car.

The therapist could not find goals upon which George and Debbie could agree. It seemed ridiculous that Debbie should have to master her fear of motorcycles in order for the marriage to succeed, but that seemed to be the only aspect on which George could focus. The therapist began to suspect that George had already decided that he wanted out of the mar-riage but was either afraid to say so or hadn't admitted it to himself yet. She began to encourage George to talk about his motorcycling despite her own reservations about the activity. The more George talked, the more it became obvious that the motorcycle riding was an overt expression of the way in which he intended to live his life. Debbie began to talk about how she didn't really want to spend her life trailing around from city to city and country to country while George chased his taste for excitement. He made no efforts to persuade her to do so. They were able to agree that their goal ought to be at least a trial separation, the terms of which they negotiated with the therapist. A follow-up interview 6 months later revealed that they had decided to remain friends but to make the separation permanent.

Help Family Members to Say What They Haven't Said, or Make Co-vert Goals Overt. There are a number of ways of making covert goals overt, depending on what people are labeling as their problem. In the case of George and Debbie, the therapist used the motorcycle as a metaphor to explore and make explicit the couple's differences. In another example, Mark and Joan came to therapy complaining that they could not get along despite months of marital therapy in another city. They had hoped things would improve after their recent move because Mark's new job involved a promotion and thus would allow them a more comfortable life-style. However, if anything, the situation had deteriorated. Although the couple complained that they could not communicate, the therapist noted that during the first two sessions, they communicated a great deal. They poured out confessions about the ways in which they had failed each other, their hopes to do better, and their despair at not succeeding despite their previ-ous therapy. In this case, the sheer volume of talk was helping them to avoid saying what was most relevant, that is that they no longer wanted to be married to each other. Their extensive communications made it possi-ble to avoid dealing with their feelings of sadness, pain, and loss. The ther-apist intervened by asking them not to talk about their relationship for one week, but to think carefully about what they wanted from each other, and whether they really wanted this marriage to continue. During the next session, each partner was able to state that they no longer wished to work on the marriage.

Anticipate the Radical Solution. In both the above cases, the therapist had some suspicion that one or both partners had already decided on the radical step of separation but wanted to do everything possible before making the move. This same wish to do everything possible before making a radical break in a relationship sometimes exists in families with difficult adolescents or young adults. Some families are so unsuccessful in their attempts to deal with gradual separation and differentiation that they come to therapy having covertly decided that the survival of the family depends on the abrupt expulsion of the young adult. The therapist should anticipate this radical solution and help the family state it openly. It is easier to cope with once it has been made a legitimate topic of discussion rather than being an anxiety-laden undercurrent.

Many therapists get caught up in the family's anxiety and conspire with family members to avoid mentioning the possibility of an impending separation. This often results in mounting tension within the family, with the problem member provoking a crisis so the other family members unite to expel him. The therapist receives a phone call announcing that the family has precipitously placed the offending member in a hospital, drug program, boarding school, or whatever type of institution they could find which would accept him/her.

Once the question of placing the adolescent or young adult is raised by the therapist, family members can talk about the pros and cons of this solution. In many cases, they may recognize that this plan is only a temporary solution to their problems, allowing the therapist to refocus on how they can cope more effectively without excluding their problem member. In other cases, placement outside the home may be necessary temporarily, but if this decision is made over time rather than in the heat of crisis, it will have fewer long-term negative effects.

Problem 6. Disagreements between the family and the therapist about the problem

Therapists and families must be able to reach some agreement about the nature of the problems on which they plan to work together. In the beginning of this chapter, it was stated that it is not necessary for the therapist to tell the family everything he/she thinks about them, nor is it necessary for all family members to agree on the specific problems and goals as long as there is agreement on more general ones. It is also not necessary for all family members to agree with the therapist about the nature of the problem, although it is always problematic when there are disagreements about central issues. Disagreements between the therapist and powerful family members, those who are in a position to either initiate change or sabotage therapy, are particularly problematic. These disagreements occur most often when parents are requesting a return to the status quo while the therapist is pushing for a meaningful change in family rules, structure or functioning. The therapist is invested in second-order change while family members are concentrating on first-order modifications. Unless the therapist can persuade the family members that a change in the way they behave toward each other will be beneficial for all of them, therapy will fail.

The Lowe family presents a good example of therapist disagreement with powerful family members about the nature of the problem. Mr. and Mrs. Lowe had married as soon as they graduated from college, had promptly had a girl and a boy, and almost had lived happily ever after. They were good people who visited their parents regularly, even when they didn't feel like it. Their peace was disturbed when their daughter, Ginnie, joined a cult in her first year of college. Eventually they literally kidnapped her and took her home where she was debriefed. The family explanation for her joining the cult was that she had been hypnotized. They then sent Ginnie to the same college her younger brother attended so that he could keep an eye on her. The family was referred when the parents discovered that Ginnie was binge eating and then forcing herself to throw up.

The Lowe's response to discovering Ginnie's binging and vomiting was to escalate their already intrusive supervision of her life. When she was home, one of them was with her constantly. When she was at school, her father called her daily, and her mother called her every couple of days. Both parents questioned her in detail about her activities, asking for reports of what she did from the time she got up in the morning until she went to bed at night. The therapist felt strongly that the Lowes had to change their overprotective parenting style before Ginnie could learn to deal with the stresses of her life in a more productive way. Her parents, however, could see no connection between their behavior and Ginnie's symptoms.

SUGGESTIONS

Join with the Parents on the Level of Their Anxiety. In the above case, the therapist told the parents that she recognized that they had been stung by Ginnie's joining a cult and that under the circumstances, their anxiety was justified. Many times family members who are insisting on their own definitions of problems become much more flexible when they feel their side of the story has been heard and respected. By spending time communicating an understanding of the fears of parents, the therapist can eventually obtain a contract which includes a more mutual problem definition and more mutual goals. Comments expressing an awareness of the anxiety inherent in having a child leave home, become symptomatic, and endanger her own life, help the family to begin to trust the therapist as someone who neither blames them nor will ask them to do more than they can tolerate. This trust in turn enables family members to be more receptive to the therapist's idea that they will eventually have to back off in order for their daughter to become independent, however difficult that may be. It also enables parents to begin to accept the reassurance that disaster will probably not result.

Even well-educated people are confused about the meaning of symptoms associated with behavioral or psychiatric disorders. Parents and siblings may be very alarmed by symptoms which appear severe but pose no immediate danger. In Ginnie's case, her parent's anxiety was heightened by recent publicity about anorexia nervosa. While it appeared that Ginnie had experienced many of the symptoms of anorexia, her current weight was stable, and her nutrition was adequate. Ginnie's parents were relieved to hear that Ginnie was in no immediate danger of starving herself.

Label the Patient's Behavior as Provocative. It is important that therapists remain in alliance with the power in the family no matter how much they may disagree with that family member's interpretation of the problem. When therapists label the patient's behavior as provocative, the implication is that the other family members are responding to provocation rather than causing the symptomatic behavior. This technique is particularly useful in joining families in which a child, adolescent, or young adult is the patient, since most parents already feel guilty and are thus sensitive that someone will blame them for their child's problems. They will trust therapists more when they don't fall into this trap. This labeling also makes other family members less vulnerable to emotional blackmail by the identified patient.

For example, the therapist also told Mr. and Mrs. Lowe that Ginnie's throwing up when she was home was an invitation to them to treat her as a much younger child, an invitation that they must resist. This moved the focus from their behavior to hers, giving them a way of seeing their behavior as connected to Ginnie's symptom without blaming them for it. The therapist did not try to communicate her belief that their excessive dependence on each other and their children, and their obsession with doing everything "right," had crippled Ginnie's ability to form appropriate relationships with her peers and handle the stress of being in college. It was enough that the therapist and Ginnie's parents could agree that there was a connection between Ginnie's symptoms and their parenting behavior.

The Negotiated Settlement. After the views of the family have been fully explored, and the views of the therapist have been explained in so far as is necessary to develop a reasonable treatment agreement, the issues separating the family and the therapist can be clarified. Once they are clarified, it is often possible to negotiate a settlement or compromise about what is to be included in the contract, even at times agreeing to disagree and still work on the problem.

Problem 7. Disagreements between the therapist and family members about goals

Therapists will often disagree with the goals of the family. Most frequently they will see the goals as too limited, too ambitious, or too vague. Some families seem to expect the moon when they come into therapy. They put inappropriate stress on becoming the perfect family, which they often equate with having no conflicts. Clearly, this goal is an unrealistic one. On the other hand, some families have no hope for improvement at all. Their goals are so limited that they see themselves as incapable of achieving any real change. Such families find it difficult to commit themselves to working in therapy. Other families have trouble defining their goals in a meaningful way, stressing pervasive discontent and vague generalities. Often these families attempt to get the therapist to set their goals. They ask the therapist what he/she thinks instead of taking some responsibility for deciding and expressing what they want.

SUGGESTIONS

If a Family Has Goals Which Are Too Ambitious, Sort Out What about Those Goals Is Possible and What Is Not. Therapists must question the realism of goals such as the elimination of conflict. While it is sometimes useful to have an ideal to strive for, believing it is attainable may cause bitterness and discouragement. In a family in which the wife's goal was for them to be more like the Waltons, the therapist discovered that this wife could not appreciate the attempts her husband made to please her because he never seemed as patient and loving as John Walton. Her ideal was self-defeating. Therapists, therefore, should always help the family to move toward the possible. This may require some education of families about what is normal family functioning. Therapists must make it clear that a certain amount of conflict, tension, and disagreement are a normal part of family life and do not imply lack of caring or love. Therapists are in unique positions to do this, since they have been exposed to the internal functioning of many families. Most people only know their own experience, and those presented in the media. As noted in this example, media views have led some families to expect the impossible and then to resent other family members when it is not available to them.

When Families Are Hopeless about Achieving Change, Set Very Small Goals. It is often necessary to break the change process down into small steps which can be seen as manageable. Families dominated by hopelessness have often been struggling with a chronic problem or a severe mental illness for a number of years and have become discouraged by their lack of progress. Therapists must help families, and themselves, to see very small achievements as significant gains. As these small gains are made, family members will perceive themselves as capable of achieving even greater changes over time. Some families have found the concept of an "internal yardstick" useful. Created by one of our expatients, this concept involves family members comparing themselves to where they were a few months ago, rather than to where other families are today. This process helps them to appreciate small signs of progress, and to build on them over time.

Expand the Focus. When families are vague about either problems or goals, or both, it is often because they are afraid to focus on the real issues. They come to therapy much like the patient who goes to his doctor complaining of vague aches and pains, certain he has a terminal condition, but afraid to be specific about what hurts for fear of what he will hear. When the doctor finds the source of pain, the patient is both afraid of the diagnosis and glad the doctor has found the problem. A classic example of this occurred when a business executive and his second wife brought their beautiful 3-year-old daughter to the Family Therapy Clinic. At the therapist's suggestion, they had left their year-old son at home. Their complaints were fairly specific; they were concerned about Lisa's apparently willful disobedience, particularly toward her mother. During this discussion, Lisa was amusing herself with puppets, but responded cheerfully when the therapist directed questions and comments to her. When questioned as to what changes they would like, they did not say they wanted to learn to control Lisa, or improve the mother–daughter relationship, but just looked helpless and confused. Finally, the father said he just wanted to know if Lisa was "okay."

The therapist avoided the mother's opening gambit of "It must be me," and began to explore the situation. In a short time, she had learned that the family recently had moved to the city from San Francisco, that Lisa's baby brother had been colicky since birth, that Lisa's mother hadn't had a good night's sleep since then, and that Lisa's father had an erratic work history. He had a pattern of being very successful for awhile and then abruptly quitting his job. Recently he had begun complaining about his current position and was threatening to quit. The tension between Lisa's parents was incredibly high, her mother alternately terrified that her husband would abandon them as he had his first family, and afraid other days that he would not. Most of this information was presented in a matter-of-fact way, as if all families lived with this level of stress. Lisa's parents were so overwhelmed with their problems that they denied them completely, leaving Lisa to become the classic conflict deviation device à la

Lynn Hoffman (1971). Broadening the focus to include the wide range of stresses on the family allowed Lisa's parents and the therapist to expand their understanding of the problems and goals, leading to a viable contract.

Narrow the Focus. Some families are vague because specifics have tended to cause fights, or because the problem has gone on so long, it seems as though everything "is wrong." With these families, it may be helpful to repeatedly ask for examples when they present generalized complaints and very vague goals. For instance, if they don't communicate, what don't they communicate about? What do they specifically want to achieve with each other? If a family is forced to repeatedly give detailed examples of what they don't like and what they would like to have happen instead, the therapist is usually able to quickly spot the underlying issues. Avram and Zahavah were a young Israeli couple, temporarily living in this country. In the first several sessions, Zahavah was very vague about her dissatisfactions and the complaints she had about Avram's behavior. She kept repeating the accusations that he put his career needs before her career needs, while Avram answered each accusation by presenting factual information about why he had to do the things she objected to in order to support the family and keep their visas. Since Zahavah knew that this was true, she would back down, only to repeat her complaint in another form. When the therapist pushed her to give very detailed examples of her complaints, it became clear that the real issue was not the priority her husband placed on his career, but that she did not feel important to him in any area. It was not a question of the amount of time he spent with her, but a question of whether any of the time he spent was quality time which made her feel relevant to his life.

Resistances to keeping contracts

The mere creation of a contract makes the entire course of treatment easier. A clear contract with specific, attainable, and mutual goals short-circuits ongoing struggles about the terms of treatment and the roles of those involved. This is not to say that the terms of a contract will not be challenged repeatedly. Family members will fail to attend sessions, will develop patterns of repeated lateness, will refuse to focus on the issues they themselves have defined as top priority. They will fail to take responsibility for change or fail to complete tasks assigned by the therapist.

The advantage of a clear contract is that it provides a guide for therapists, and a method by which they retain control of the process of treatment. Each time a therapist encounters new behaviors, new topics, or inexplicable responses, he/she can ask himself/herself and the family,

"How does this relate to our contract? Is this something we agreed to work on?" If it fits with the contract, well and good. If it does not, the therapist has two options: He/she can refocus on the terms of the existing contract or initiate a discussion to revise the contract or create a new one.

For instance, if a family begins to come sporadically, a therapist reminds the family that the agreement was for 12 weekly sessions. If the family brings up new, and seemingly less important issues, a therapist can point out that the family had established x and y as their priorities, thereby returning to the original focus. If the new issue, z, actually sounds more relevant than x and y, the therapist can suggest that the contract be revised to make z the focus. For example, a therapist can say, "Although we agreed to focus on x, this issue sounds much more important to all of you, what about if we agree to do this first, and then return to x?"

Keeping the contract in mind is of great value, particularly to beginners. Most beginners are uncomfortable with the use of their own power, and taking active control of sessions. A contract enables them to place the burden of control on the agreement. Therapists become the enforcers of what the family has said they wanted and/or of what they have already committed themselves to. Although lapses from the contract may still occur, if therapists are clear about the rules and direction of treatment, they can more easily evaluate the significance of these lapses.

In effective contract enforcement, as in all family therapy, sequences and patterns of behavior are most important. Therefore, in evaluating a particular resistance to the contract, the principle to remember is to evaluate it within the context of the contract. Some lapses from the contract may be ignored by the therapist in the service of achieving long-term goals. However, consistent lapses on the part of the most resistant family members cannot be ignored if those goals are to be reached. To return to the example of Jason, Jon, and Sarah, Jason's noncompliance could be minimized for quite some time as long as Sarah and Jon were keeping their part of the contract consistently. The therapist knew that eventually Jason would have to come to terms with the new behaviors of his parents.

Problem 1. Failure of one or all members to attend regularly as promised

The most obvious overt resistances to the contract are broken appointments and lateness. Families who call to cancel or reschedule appointments, families who consistently fail to attend but respond to the therapist's inquiries with statements of good intentions, and families who are consistently late are all examples of this form of resistance. These problems are easier to combat in the contract maintenance phase of treatment if therapists have been able to develop a clear contract early on. If so, they have at least a verbal commitment to the basic rules of treatment, and presumably they also have had time to establish a relationship with powerful family members (see also Chapter 2).

SUGGESTIONS

Evaluate the Therapist's Own Behavior. Remember, every behavior must be evaluated within the context of what is happening within the family and within the therapy. If one member has agreed to come, but suddenly begins missing sessions, the therapist may want to review his/her interventions to see if he/she has unwittingly allied with other family members or has neglected the needs of the abstainer in some important way. If this proves to be true, the therapist can either make the issue explicit, admitting to an error and asking to be called on it if it occurs again, or they can simply attend to the person's needs more carefully in future sessions.

If recalcitrant family members have serious negative reactions to the therapist or the sessions, these reactions are best discussed openly. However, family members usually must be encouraged to give feedback and speak out. If the person(s) is distressed by the therapist's style, perhaps the therapist can modify it. If the objections are impossible to overcome, there is nothing wrong with offering another therapist. Not every therapist is for every family. Often family members will refuse the offer of another therapist, but the offer having been made can give them the feeling that their complaints have been understood and taken seriously, enabling them to begin to work more earnestly with the current one.

Send a Personal Invitation. The therapist may find it necessary to go out of his/her way to reinvolve someone who has disengaged from therapy. He/she may call the refuser, elicit the practical problems involved with attendance, and negotiate with him/her directly, using statements which emphasize the member's importance, such as "I don't think we're going to get anywhere without you." Even when family members are bent on avoiding the pain of therapy sessions, they are often flattered and interested when the therapist takes time to reach out to them in this way.

Help the Family to Reinvolve the Resister(s). Following the principle of keeping as much responsibility in the family as possible, the therapist can make the absence of certain members a subject of the family sessions. Not only can the family be given strategies by the therapist which have worked with other families engaged in such struggles, but they can also be asked to brainstorm to come up with ideas which will bring the absent members back. The parents in one family described in the literature decided to retain a part of their son's allowance if he did not come to therapy, because they believed his absence was likely to make the therapy last longer, and, therefore, be more expensive for the family. A variety of such strategies can be shared with the family, while encouraging them to come up with their own special techniques based on what they know about one another.

It is best to discourage parents from using outright bribery, which is a relatively ineffective technique that often has negative side effects. Parents who use this strategy usually do so because they feel they have little effective control over their children. For instance, one mother bribed her son to come to therapy, thus knowingly supplying him with the money which fed his habit of abusing cough medicine. In such situations, the therapist should attempt to help the family to find some other strategy for gaining cooperation. In this case, the therapist was able to encourage the boy's father to take over the job of enforcing attendance at therapy, and he was able to do so effectively.

Offer Fewer Sessions. It may be easier to get a resistant member to agree to monthly therapy sessions when weekly sessions are unacceptable. Selvini Palazzoli and her colleagues (1978) claim to have had excellent results with this frequency, but this response may be specific to their highly specialized approach. Nevertheless, it is worth a try and therapists should evaluate the possible advantages and disadvantages of infrequent appointments versus the possibility of losing one or more family members altogether. Like Selvini Palazzoli, they may find that what began as a necessity, becomes an advantage. However, therapists should examine their motives before instituting this plan. They must not use it simply to avoid taking a stand with a family, or as a way of avoiding their own anxiety about family sessions. The strategy should only be used when therapists believe they can accomplish something on a monthly basis.

Problem 2. Failure to perform assigned tasks

Many family therapists use tasks to achieve their goals, whether the tasks are designed to restructure the family, reinforce changes discussed in sessions, or create a situation which causes spontaneous change to occur within the family. Tasks can be as specific as "Joe will take out the garbage every other day and father will be in charge of making sure that he does," or as vague as "Sarah will help Jon deal with Jason," depending on what the therapist wishes to achieve. In general, the more specific the task, the easier it is for the family to do, and the easier it is for the therapist to decide whether or not it has been accomplished. While it is easy to determine whether Joe took out the garbage, it is harder to determine if Sarah helped Jon deal with Jason. The latter is a judgment call.

Tasks are extremely useful but compliance by family members is often a problem. The therapist must establish some power within the family before he/she can hope to gain the family's cooperation in following through with tasks. Although simply being labeled, "the therapist," is enough to inspire some cooperation, it is sometimes necessary to emphasize the therapist's expertise or the usefulness of tasks. Failure to perform tasks is always a resistance. The resistance, however, may well be caused by therapist error. Many therapists, particularly new ones, assign tasks that are far too ambitious or that are not immediately relevant to the problem as the family sees it.

SUGGESTIONS

Evaluate the Task. Before taking other steps, it is important to question family members to determine whether therapist error is to blame for the family's failure to follow through on the assignment. During this discussion the therapist must ask himself/herself, "Considering this family's way of operating, how difficult was this task?" In other words, the therapist assesses whether the task was too ambitious for the family, or whether he/she lacked the leverage to gain compliance. The therapist should review the task with the family to discover the specific reasons that it was not completed, using their account of why the task was not done, diagnostically. Their level of resistance can be easily discerned while gathering additional data about the family's organization and interactional patterns in the process. The discussion about the task and the circumstances surrounding their noncompliance places an emphasis upon the task which reinforces the importance the therapist attaches to it. Usually, after conducting the task review, therapists will find the task was too vague or impossibly ambitious, but this, too, gives them valuable information to use in making future assignments. Recently, for instance, one of our interns asked a very estranged couple to spend an hour each evening talking about their relationship. The couple did so for about 15 minutes the first night, got into a huge argument, didn't speak for the rest of the week, and came to the next session on the verge of a divorce. The therapist realized he had assigned a task which was impossible for a couple who had not yet decided if they even wanted to talk.

If therapists determine that they have made an error, that is, if they have assigned a task that was too difficult or not relevant, they should admit it. Although some experts, Jay Haley, for instance, have stated that therapists should hold families responsible for their failures to perform tasks (Haley, 1976), it seems likely that there are clear advantages to admitting errors in task assignment. Therapists not only enhance their credibility by freely admitting that a task was wrong and assigning a more appropriate one, but they also avoid making the family feel badly about themselves for being unable to accomplish something so seemingly easy.

Reassign the Same Task. If the evaluation of the task leads to the conclusion that it was both relevant and appropriate, the therapist should ask the family to try it again. The family may be testing the therapist to see how seriously they should take instructions, or they may be displaying their own ambivalence about change. Reassigning a task underlines and reinforces its importance and the importance of following through on therapeutic directives. Small variations in the prescription of the task can be made if the variation will help family members to save face, or if it enhances chances that the task will be performed without interfering with its original purpose.

Assign an Easier or More Specific Task. If therapists would like to use tasks, they should not give up the idea just because one has failed. Dropping the assignment gives the family the impression that the therapist is inconsistent; or isn't to be taken seriously. If therapists don't follow through, they may find increased problems with family compliance on other issues. Furthermore, enough is learned by examining the failure of a task to make it possible to create and assign a more appropriate one.

In the couple described above, an appropriate task would probably be a far more limited one. For instance, they might have been asked to set aside a half-hour once during the week to talk about an activity they would enjoy doing together. This limits both the subject and the time, thus avoiding pressures and intimacies they are not yet ready to handle. While most couples and families will balk slightly at tasks that sound easy ("That's no problem, we can do more"), tasks are always more difficult than they seem.

This is not to say that families can never tolerate difficult tasks. Sometimes they can rise to the challenge. One of our residents recently encountered a large, noisy, disorganized family in which everyone complained about everyone else's behavior. The parents were totally unable to establish reasonable expectations for compliance around simple household matters. The resident was a highly organized fellow himself. The confusion of the family session was more than he could tolerate, so, against his supervisor's advice, he limited the sessions to seeing only the parents. Then, also against his supervisor's advice, he worked out a complicated system of rules for the parents to establish at home with fines for noncompliance. Amazingly, the parents were not only able to keep the task straight but they collected fines from their children and took themselves out on Saturday night using their accumulated funds.

Give Them a Choice of Another Task. It sometimes helps to give the family a choice of repeating the previous task or receiving another one which is similarly structured but puts the onus for change on another family member. Change is never symmetrical and simultaneous in any system. Usually some parts of the system are ready to move before others. If one family member is somewhat more ready to move than another, there is no point in struggling with the more resistant one. In the interest of conserving therapist energy and avoiding therapist fatigue, it is a good principle to follow the line of least resistance. Giving the family a choice of tasks can be diagnostic in determining who is ready to move within the system, and also minimizes resistance by emphasizing their sense of control over the process. Furthermore, it can encourage a little healthy competition between family members as to who is "most ready" and "most cooperative."

The Carlson family included two very resistant adolescent girls. Neither wanted to come to therapy, much less participate in the discussions or follow through on tasks. When the girls blatantly refused to do a task, the therapist said this was perfectly all right, that they were not ready to make changes in the family. She went on to describe the parents as more invested in change as this point. They were asked to spend some time together discussing and coming to some agreement on one or two rules for their daughters. When they returned the following week, not only had the parents completed their task, but the girls had completed the task that had been discussed but not assigned to them.

Use a Paradoxical Message. The above suggestion is in some ways a paradoxical technique, a method that can be used more generally. If a relevant and meaningful task has not been performed and the therapist believes that it has not been completed because the family is directly resisting either the therapist or change, the therapist may find a paradoxical message the intervention of choice. The therapist can label change as dangerous, or the family as moving too fast, urging the family to abandon the task or supporting their resistance to it. If the family does abandon the task, the therapist is still in charge, having told them to do so. If they choose to "defeat" the therapist by completing the task, they will have made a change for the better. For example, a psychiatrist referred a boutique owner and his wife to the Family Therapy Clinic because the doctor was concerned about the symbiotic relationship between the mother, whom he was treating for chronic severe depression, and her 10-year-old daughter. The couple complained that they could not get their daughter to stay in her own bed at night. Each night, the child complained that she could not sleep and she would creep into her parents' bed. When the therapist questioned this practice, the mother claimed she could not bear to think of her daughter lying awake, all alone. Besides, she complained, because of her medication she was always too soundly asleep to notice when the child came into their bed. The father stated he could not carry the child back to her own bed because of his bad back, and she simply would not go back on her own. The couple consistently resisted the obvious simple solution of locking their bedroom door. The therapist began to take the position that they were absolutely right, that there must be something unreasonable about asking a 10-year-old to sleep in her own bed, and speculating about how big a bed they would need when she grew into adolescence.

After a few weeks of this, the father abruptly locked the bedroom door, ordering his daughter back to her bedroom when she repeatedly knocked on the door. After several nights, the little girl ceased knocking on the door.

Problem 3. The wrong focus

The family that neglects to bring up a very important issue is very much like the family that fails to mention a very important person. Family members may collude to cover up a sensitive issue, often fearing that it will blow the family apart or hurt others too deeply. If therapists do not discover the issue on their own initiative, their interventions mysteriously fail, and they are left to wonder why the contract is not working. This form of resistance is particularly common in families in which there has been some sexual involvement, real or imagined, between an adolescent and a parent, stepparent, or parental consort. In such families, all members are usually in a covert alliance to cover up the sexual activity, either out of guilt or fear of breaking up the family.

When family members have colluded to avoid sharing a real issue with the therapist, it may not be a conscious decision made by family members, but rather an adherence to unconscious family rules about not talking about certain subjects, or not criticizing certain members. In some cases, one real issue is used to avoid a focus on another more painful one. All family therapists, sooner or later, encounter the classic example of this phenomenon, that in which a family persists in focusing on the symptoms of the identified patient in order to avoid dealing with a painful conflict between the parents. In one recent case, a young girl named Lilly had fits of uncontrollable vomiting which left her exhausted and gasping for breath. The family's focus on this hideous symptom was understandable. Lilly's parents could not understand why anyone would recommend family therapy. They insisted that their family was perfect, going on to explain that they had only had two arguments in their 22 years of marriage. This lack of conflict was remarkable in view of the differences between them. Lilly's father was lean, demanding, perfectionistic, and extremely controlling. He openly stated his children were welcome to live in his house until they were 35, as long as they did things his way. Lilly's mother was plump and easygoing. She never quite managed to keep the house up to her husband's perfectionistic standards. In fact, recently she hardly did any housework at all. Lilly did most of it, hating the fact that it prevented her from spending time with her friends, but terrified that her father would explode if he found the house a mess. Yet, when her father ventured that maybe he demanded too much from his daughter, both Lilly and her mother reassured him that his standards were reasonable. When Lilly suggested her mother could do more of the housework, the father defended his wife, claiming she needed a little leisure time. Lilly quickly agreed and, smiling inappropriately, sank into silence. The obvious differences between the parents were either denied or joked about by all family members, while Lilly remained stuck in the middle. The only way she could get out of the housework and yet avoid responsibility for maintaining peace in the family was to develop a debilitating symptom. The therapist, caught up in sympathy for Lilly, suggested that there was an inherent conflict between father's demands and mother's behavior. The entire family attacked the therapist and subsequently dropped out of treatment, claiming that after five sessions, Lilly only threw up on days they had a family therapy appointment, so clearly it was family therapy that was disturbing her.

It isn't only "perfect" families that collude to deny important topics. Family members may be openly hostile to each other and yet collude to avoid discussing a crucial issue. The family of a young woman named Dorothy illustrates this phenomenon. She came to therapy with her mother and her three younger sisters. Her open rebellion against her mother was the presenting complaint. It quickly developed that she was also openly hostile to her mother's boyfriend who had moved in and was apparently trying to establish himself as a source of authority. At the therapist's suggestion, the boyfriend, Rob, was included in the therapy. Dorothy's mother consistently supported Rob's efforts to control the children in what looked like a good attempt to establish a parental coalition and firm generational boundaries. Despite increased consistency and what seemed to be good will, things did not improve. The situation became increasingly dangerous when Dorothy began to repeatedly provoke Rob into open physical fights resulting in minor injuries. When the therapist finally saw Dorothy alone, she blurted out an accusation that Rob had tried to sexually molest her while her mother was in the hospital having a hysterectomy. Filled with guilt, and fearful that if her mother knew she would reject her and take Rob's side, she had kept her secret. What she could not keep secret was her overwhelming anger at her mother for not protecting her and at Rob for taking advantage of her. She felt both she and Rob had betrayed her mother.

SUGGESTIONS

Don't Precipitate a Confrontation Too Quickly. It's useful to remember that people are extremely sensitive about whatever it is they are working so hard to ignore. If a family does not bring up an issue spontaneously, chances are there is an unspoken rule about not doing so. Pointing out sensitive issues, particularly in an early interview, may result in families terminating prematurely as in Lilly's case, and the case of the resident who allowed the discussion of parenting problems to proceed into a discussion of marital problems too quickly. Timing is absolutely crucial, as is the way in which the confrontation is framed. It is best to wait until the therapist has developed at least a little trust, and then to try a tentative intervention to test the waters. If the toe says the waters are too cold, it's best not to do a full body plunge.

Relabel Issues. If Lilly's therapist, a senior clinician, had been a little less caught up in her sympathy with Lilly's desperate struggle for control over her own life, she might have kept the case by relabeling the conflict between Lilly's parents as representing the normal tensions between different, complimentary, people. When conflict has been labeled as normal, it is less threatening to discuss. The problem could then have been defined as finding some way to help Lilly establish some control over her vomiting by staying out of her parents normal disagreements and establishing some control over other aspects of her life.

Be Prepared for Anxiety and Attacks on the Therapist. It is sometimes necessary to confront sensitive issues directly, even when this action might result in a family dropping out of treatment. In extremely resistant families where nothing else has worked, and where the risk is worth it to achieve quick change or prevent impending disaster, therapists can confront sensitive issues directly. However, such therapists must be able to tolerate family members' anxiety and even their angry attacks. For example, in a case referred from an inpatient unit Joel, a 9-year-old boy, had threatened to kill himself and had set the family's house on fire. His parents refused to take any responsibility either for Joel's disturbance or for making any changes in the way the family functioned. They persistently complained about the school not placing Joel in the right class. Despite the resistance he knew he would encounter, the therapist confronted them with their hopelessly inadequate parenting and their excessive drinking. They became very defensive and attacked the therapist who simply kept repeating his statement that they had to do something quickly because their son was completely out of control. Joel's parents missed the next two sessions but the therapist persisted in calling them and restating his point. He also mobilized other systems to join in his attempt to engage them in constructive action. Eventually they came in and made modest efforts at changing their parenting. These direct confrontations are very difficult for therapists who do not work in a supportive context, and thus are recommended for those in private practice only when they are feeling both courageous and energetic.

Problem 4. An inconsistent focus

Keeping a dialogue or family discussion going in one direction until something has been resolved or agreed upon is often very difficult. This is particularly true because families are usually discussing what they find most uncomfortable, and therefore any escape is welcome. In a variation of the bait-and-switch approach so popular with appliance stores, families may come with a new problem every week to avoid discussing the primary one for which they came to treatment. The new problem is described as infinitely more pressing and more interesting than the old one. These new problems may be introduced as a new crisis or as something the therapist should have discovered weeks ago.

This was true of the socially prominent Sands family. They and their three children were handsome and well dressed. During the first few weeks of therapy they talked about the oldest son's drug abuse. Next they discussed the second son's persistent lying. The father was fond of presenting the newest problem or crisis with a slight hint of sarcasm, intimating that the therapist should have been able to predict or prevent the newest crisis. He started off each session with "Well, you know Jeffrey's been expelled for lying again," or "Of course, you can guess that John got drunk and wrecked the car." An unspoken "And what are you going to do about it?" hung in the air. When the therapist attempted to focus on the need for a stronger, more coherent parental coalition, the parents presented some other disastrous problem, or one of the children provoked a crisis. The therapist was sure the marital alliance was in shambles, but both parents claimed they would be happily married if it weren't for their dreadful children. The therapist allowed them to keep the focus on their children, but kept insisting they make a coherent set of rules and enforce them. She was not surprised when they reacted by putting their oldest son into individual therapy the next time he provoked a crisis. Nor was she surprised when a year later, the father attempted suicide and they finally returned for marital therapy.

SUGGESTIONS

Focus on the Lack of Focus. The contract itself can be used to control the lack of focus. When each new issue arises, the therapist can comment that it is not a part of the current contract. If the family feels an issue is sufficiently important to take precedence over the other issues they have defined as priorities, then the contract is renegotiated explicitly. Usually, if the new issue is a resistance, the question about its significance is sufficient to refocus on the real business of the session.

Some families, however, are chaotic. The raising and dropping of issues without resolution has become a way of life. Their inability to focus and therefore to resolve problems, must become one of the problems on which they contract to work. Once the significance of this issue has been established, whole sessions can be structured around helping them to reach agreement about an issue or about a task to be performed in the coming week. Progress can be measured by the length of time it takes them to complete a transaction over the course of therapy. One family recently took an excruciating 1 hour and 20 minutes to reach their first decision. Everyone had to volunteer several suggestions and interrupt everyone else at least twice. By the end of treatment, only 3 or 4 minutes were required to reach a decision.

Ignore the Change and Pursue Your Focus. If the change in focus is clearly an attempt to avoid a painful issue, the therapist can deal with the new issue for a time and then return to the painful one, or she/he can simply block the family's attempt to change the focus. The Wilsons were a single-parent family who came to treatment because the mother felt she could not control her rebellious children. Some progress was made in establishing rules and expectations, but soon they reached a point in treatment where it became clear that they had to deal with their feelings about the father's death. Their feelings about the father/husband, and the way he died, were making it difficult to be a family, yet his death had never been discussed or mourned as a family. When bits and pieces of information about the father began to come out toward the end of a session, family members reluctantly agreed that the issue of mourning must now be discussed. The next session began with a huge crisis. One of the adolescent girls said she could no longer live in the family. One of the boys overturned a table and ran out of the room. The mother angrily stated that the only way that the therapist could help her was by finding a suitable boarding school for her three children because she just couldn't take it anymore. After asking one family member to retrieve the boy who had bolted from the room, the therapist did not deal with the crisis because she thought it was a red herring. She went straight to the issue of the loss. "I guess it's a lot easier to fight with one another than to talk about how sad you feel and how much you miss your husband/father." Nearly everyone began to cry at once, and the process of mourning had begun.

Put the Responsibility for Change on Them. Families are often adept at inducing a therapist to take all the responsibility for change, nearly as adept as therapists are at taking too much responsibility and running with it. Not adhering to a consistent focus is one way of not taking responsibility. Asking the family to police its own tendencies to bring up new subjects, and teaching them some techniques for doing so, puts the responsibility on them to decide how they are going to use the session. A professor and his wife and son were referred to the Family Therapy Clinic after the son was arrested on charges of attempted rape. In fact, he had not so much attempted rape as he had just hung around outside the homes of some adolescent girls and tried to touch their breasts and buttocks and then run away. The parents were shocked and frightened, particularly by the police involvement. They were quite ready to make a contract to begin setting limits on their son's behavior, something they had not done before. However, as soon as the immediate danger of a trial was over, all three family members began losing track of the subject being discussed in therapy, interrupting each other frequently. The therapist pointed out that now that the charges had been dropped everyone seemed less interested in pursuing the contract. All three admitted they were feeling less tense, but also said this was pretty much how things went at home, nothing ever got quite resolved. The therapist then asked each one to try to keep a focus on the issue being discussed, to refrain from interrupting anyone else, and to start each sentence with "I think." The family had an experience of exchanging ideas, all trying hard to take responsibility for not interrupting anyone else and for reaching a conclusion to their discussion.

Label the Session a Holiday. If some change has been achieved in the past but now the family seems to be wandering, it is sometimes wise to declare the session a holiday and spend the time "socializing" with them. If a therapist uses this technique, it is important that he/she label the behavior so that family members do not confuse working and playing. While the wandering may well be a resistance or a reaction to something that has happened in therapy, letting the resistance serve its function and run its course is not always a bad idea. This, of course, is only appropriate when used sparingly and when the family has a history of work toward change.

For example, a family had been seen in the Family Therapy Clinic for some months. During that time, the animosity between the mother and the oldest daughter had decreased greatly and the marital situation had improved. Some problems remained, particularly in that the mother had periods of depression which seemed unrelated to family interaction. The therapist wanted to discuss this with the whole family so that the children would better understand their mother's unpredictable behavior. They would have none of it. Everyone kept changing the subject or telling the therapist stories about school. She finally gave up and said, "Since no one wants to talk about mother's depression, I'm just going to stop working so hard and let you amuse me." The family continued to amuse her for awhile, and then spontaneously returned to business.

Resistances to terminating contracts

The amount of resistance to terminating a treatment contract in family therapy varies considerably, although it is usually not a highly problematic issue for a number of reasons. In most cases, even prolonged family therapy does not involve as intense a relationship and as intense a transference as is established in traditional individual therapy. The mere presence of actual family members in the sessions leads to a focus on resolving here and now issues with real people, or at most resolving how past attachments and past learned behaviors are being inappropriately applied to current life relationships. The intensity of attachment to the therapist also is often purposefully muted by the therapist who redirects the focus to the interaction between family members rather than to a focus on the interaction with the therapist. Furthermore, some models of family therapy stress the fact that the therapist should always give credit and responsibility for change or improvement to the family rather than placing themselves in a central role and encouraging family members to become dependent on them. Finally, much family therapy is relatively short term and problem focused, thereby discouraging the development of strong dependency on the therapist.

Nevertheless, many families resist termination when it is impending. If therapy has been prolonged, and the therapist has been effective in joining the family and effecting change, he/she may be regarded almost as a family member. If families tend to be enmeshed, separation and loss are always difficult. Regardless of how skillful the therapist has been at attributing the credit for change to family members, a family will feel some degree of dependence on the therapist, and some fear of how well they will do on their own.

Again, a clear explicit contract goes a long way toward avoiding some of the problems of this phase of treatment. With a clear contract, termination becomes an almost matter-of-fact phenomenon. If a family has known from the very beginning of treatment that it will be over after 12 sessions or 6 months, they are prepared for that fact and will have invested themselves accordingly. Even if no specific number of sessions has been mentioned, if a family has known therapy will be over when goals x and y were accomplished, they usually are satisfied to stop when those goals are attained. Treatment contracts help to avoid infantilization and the inappropriate expectation that the therapist will be available ad infinitum.

The problems that arise around the issue of contract termination fall into three categories: symptom reemergence, honeymoons, and total avoidance of the issue.

Problem 1. Symptoms reemerge

Around the time the idea of termination has been raised, some family members start having the same old problems that brought them to therapy and have long since been eliminated. Old patterns of behavior and interaction suddenly reappear. Other families may begin discussions about how they fear symptoms will return, at times creating a self-fulfilling prophecy.

A family which has been functioning perfectly well on their own may suddenly start making telephone calls to the therapist between sessions or having inexplicable crises which require extra sessions. All of these phenomena are, of course, more common when the presenting problem was a very serious one and treatment was prolonged. In one family, family therapy was initiated when the failure of multiple treatments and hospitalizations over a 7-year period failed to alter the psychotic and dysfunctional behavior of a family's youngest son. After a year and a half of family treatment, the son was relatively stable, involved in social activities, and doing volunteer work at a local nonprofit organization. When the therapist moved to terminate, thinking about as much as possible had been accomplished, the boy's mother began following the boy around the house, saying, "I know you're going to get sick again." Naturally, a crisis was precipitated.

SUGGESTIONS

Call Them on Their Resistance. A therapist may explicitly connect the reemergence of symptomatic behaviors with termination. He/she may say something along the lines of "Well, I guess we can't quit yet. You're obviously telling me you're not ready." Most people deny that this is what is on their minds, and then have to prove it by managing better without the therapist. This technique works best with families that really do believe they can cope and are just a little fearful of doing so. While it would not have worked in the above example, it worked beautifully with Mary and Joe. They were referred for couples therapy after Mary suffered a bout of depression which responded nicely to antidepressant medication. However, during her depression, Mary had become very dependent on Joe and had developed a number of symptoms which made it necessary for him to be available to her at all times. These were mostly psychosomatic in nature, such as fainting spells, splitting headaches, and an occasional panic attack. These symptoms were associated with buses, stores, crossing streets, and staying home alone at night. Joe's whole business schedule had been changed so that he could take her to and from work, take her shopping, and avoid leaving her alone at night. Joe was easy going and used to a moderate amount of dependency in the 27 years he had been married to Mary, so he didn't object. Through a series of tasks and with a lot of support, Mary gradually gave up her symptoms. After a triumphant trip to California (she had been afraid of flying too) during which she spent periods of time alone in a strange city, the therapist thought termination was in order. Mary looked dismayed, and the following week telephoned the therapist to say she was leaving work because she had developed a headache. During the next session, she mentioned some minor anxiety she had felt staying home alone one night, and how she had gone next door to a neighbor for reassurance. The therapist confronted her, "Okay, Mary, if you're not ready, you're not ready. But enough of this penny-ante stuff. How about a really big regression? Joe, you better start taking her to work again and, Mary, I'd stay out of stores if I were you." There were no telephone calls between the next two appointments and Mary became less symptomatic and allowed termination to take place. She keeps in touch, sending the therapist postcards whenever she takes a trip.

Gradually Increase the Time between Sessions. Far more appropriate for the family with a seriously disturbed member is the technique of gradually weaning them from therapy. Sessions may move from every week to every fortnight, to every month, followed by 6-month checkups. In this way, the family learns they can manage on their own without ever having actually dealt with termination. It may, in fact, be unclear to everyone exactly when termination occurs. This method of gradual termination can be easier on the therapist as well. In cases where treatment has been extensive, a therapist is often invested in the success of the family at maintaining their gains. Gradually increasing the time between sessions also gives the therapist an opportunity to observe the family functioning well without constant therapeutic input, and reassures the therapist that the family can live without him/her. One of the authors treated a family in which the 26-year-old daughter had a severe eating disorder of many years' duration. Treatment was extensive and prolonged, but successful. The family and the identified patient were quite pleased with the results, leaving only the therapist fearing relapse. Sessions were gradually diminished in number until they tapered off completely. The therapist made a deal with an amused family that whenever her anxiety rate about the patient rose to an intolerable level, the family would come in so she could see for herself that they were still doing well.

Keep an Open Door. Whether families terminate clearly, or in the above fashion, it often helps them to do so more comfortably if they feel they can return if necessary. Therapists, therefore, should assure families that they can come back for a refresher course if things go sour again. Harriet and Michael came to therapy even before they were married. They both had been married before and now they were about to become a blended family, with four children between them. They used a 12-session contract very productively, anticipating problems they would encounter and setting up rules for living together. A year after the marriage, they returned for a brief time when one of their adolescent sons was acting out and skipping school. Three years later another rocky time occurred around the emancipation of a daughter. Each time the family returned for treatment they used the sessions well. Each time they seemed able to go a little longer on their own. While this particular family knew when to ask for help, sometimes it helps to teach families the signals that indicate the time has come. This helps to avoid the family letting the situation deteriorate to the point that a whole new course of therapy is necessary.

Make the Feelings Explicit. Sometimes the fears of terminating are more difficult to tolerate because they are not really fully conscious. Some ominous cloud seems to be hanging over the family and threatening its members. In these cases, the therapist can encourage them to talk about their ambivalence regarding termination and their fears about ending therapy. This process, combined with reassurances that the therapist thinks the family is ready, is often enough.

Focus on Strengths. At the end of therapy, it is good to review what the family has accomplished, stressing what they have learned about one another, about problem solving, and about how to cope. Placing an emphasis on their strengths and abilities while providing some sort of cognitive distance on the experience of therapy helps to provide the closure needed to leave therapy comfortably. Many families seem surprised when they look back over the course of therapy and see how far they have come. While it would be tempting for a therapist to take the credit, it is important to attribute these gains to the family's own work and abilities, giving them confidence they can do it on their own in the future.

Problem 2. Honeymoons

Another method families use to avoid dealing with termination realistically is to create a "love in" atmosphere. Not only do they describe their family and their relationships as wonderful, but the therapist is wonderful, too. It is tempting for a therapist to agree with such a family, particularly when it means that the therapist can pat himself/herself on the back and take credit for the phenomenon. Rarely does one get a chance to watch a family walk smiling into a rosy sunset to live happily ever after. However, this is *not* a good way to terminate, but a resistance to dealing with termination. Terminations need not involve mourning, misery, and gnashing of teeth, but they should be realistic.

SUGGESTIONS

Review the Presenting Complaint and the Course of Treatment. Looking at what brought the family to treatment helps to add a note of reality to the termination process. It helps further to discuss the course of therapy and how they would deal with the same problem if it occurred today. Discussions of these issues help to put both good and bad feelings into perspective, and to provide some distance about an emotional experience at an emotional time. Reviewing treatment helps people to see that there were pros and cons to the treatment as well.

Predict Future Problems. No family, even one well "therapized," will continue for long without encountering some problems. Therapists can help families to cope with the inevitable emergence of problems by predicting that such problems will arise, and describing this as normal and inevitable. At the same time, they can help families to plan methods of coping with future problems in advance.

In the case of Mary and Joe, for instance, the therapist might well predict that Mary would become more phobic whenever anything happened to make her more anxious or which would disturb the family equilibrium. Both partners could be given some strategies for cooling things down, and for assessing when the signals were serious enough to ask for help again.

Problem 3. Total avoidance of the issue

Some families and therapists become so involved with one another that they fail to see that it is time to terminate. Total avoidance of the issue of termination is only possible with the therapist's collusion. Therapists who have several resistant and uncooperative families are vulnerable to hanging onto a family that is doing well, is fun to work with, and likes to come in. One of our colleagues recently described her problem letting go of such a family, saying, "It's so rare to be valued and appreciated, I hate to see them terminate." Not surprisingly, this means that some people get more therapy than they need, particularly if the therapist isn't busy. One student, for instance, just couldn't let go of her first successful case, despite the fact that things had been going well for some time.

SUGGESTIONS

Conduct a Periodic Review of the Contract. Therapists who make it a policy to periodically review the contract will always know if they have begun colluding with a family to avoid termination. Such reviews may cause therapists to discover that original goals have been reached but that their overinvolvement with the family has prevented them from seeing the need for termination. Periodic contract reviews are particularly important for therapists who are aware that they have a tendency to become overinvolved and lose their perspective.

Get Consultation. When therapists find themselves unsure if they are continuing to meet with a family because of the family's needs or their own, it is time to get some outside input. A supervisor or family therapy consultant frequently can put the situation in perspective and offer suggestions for effecting termination. If no such consultant is available, discussing a case with a colleague may help to establish some distance.

Some therapists find it helpful to establish a peer group supervision process which can provide consultation as necessary. This is particularly useful in agencies and institutions where the practice of family therapy has been only recently initiated. Since it is easy for therapists to criticize each other's work, particularly with hindsight, it may be helpful to establish a rule in such groups that each criticism be accompanied by a helpful suggestion. This helps to establish a supportive and thoughtful climate which in turn makes it easier to bring cases for consultation.

Summary

A solid and consistent treatment contract based on mutual and attainable goals is the best guarantee of success in family therapy. A treatment contract consists of all those behaviors of the therapist and family members which operate to establish the rules by which therapy will be conducted, the goals toward which the therapy is directed, and the means by which those goals will be reached. A treatment contract may be explicit or implicit but no therapist can avoid having one; it arises out of the process of therapy. It is important that all therapists realize that there is a contract process and that their behavior constantly impacts on the terms of the contract. It is particularly important that beginners make this process explicit, since it will contribute to their ability to control the direction and process of therapy.

The simplest contract agreements are around the boundaries of therapy, the question of who will come and how frequent the sessions will be. More complicated negotiations include the process of problem definition and goal setting.

The most common problems arising in the process of contract formation center on the unavailability of the whole family, the unavailability of key family members for sessions, and the differing views of problems and goals among family members or between the family and the therapist. Resistances to contract maintenance include challenges to the boundaries of therapy such as attendance and frequency of sessions, and to the work of therapy such as task completion and problems with focus. Termination resistances take the form of the reemergence of symptoms, the honeymoon phenomenon, and the collusion of therapist and family to avoid termination.

4. Challenges to the therapist's competence

> I was gratified to be able to answer promptly, and I did. I
> said I didn't know.—Mark Twain

Direct or indirect challenges to the therapist's competence can become the most destructive forms of resistance to family therapy. They can become destructive because they often start an escalating process between the family and the therapist which exacerbates the defensiveness of both. When an obviously successful middle-aged father makes an offhand comment on a therapist's youthful appearance, the therapist is likely to feel attacked. Never mind that the father has his own problems with a midlife crisis, or that he envies the therapist's easy way of relating to his adolescent son, the therapist *feels* that his/her competence is being challenged. The therapist in turn may need to prove his/her power and authority to a father very much in need of support and reassurance rather than one more power struggle. Thus, a battle is begun which will at least make therapy more difficult, and may even destroy the possibility that it can occur.

Beginning therapists are particularly vulnerable to being caught in these negative interactions. Already unsure of themselves, beginners are easily convinced that family members are absolutely right when they express reservations about the therapist's ability to help them. More experienced therapists also have their weak spots; having lived and practiced longer, they have had longer to make mistakes.

Families and therapists have particular difficulty dealing with the issue of therapist competence in part because both have mistaken or unrealistic assumptions about what constitutes competence in a family therapist. Most families tend to assume that a good therapist is one who "has it all together," personally and professionally. Most therapists, particularly those who lack experience, assume that they have to be able to answer all questions and resolve all problems immediately, or they are not good therapists. Therapists who hold such unrealistic assumptions are more likely to wilt or become defensive in the face of natural challenges by families. Unlike Mark Twain, they cannot admit to any flaw for fear of appearing incompetent. This fear is transmitted to families, inadvertently indicating there might be good reason to wonder about the therapist's abilities, and actually stimulating or exacerbating family resistance. As Napoleon said, "He who fears being conquered is sure of defeat."

This is not to say that some family members don't deliberately raise questions about the therapist's qualifications in order to avoid a focus on their own behaviors. In some cases a challenge to the therapist's competence serves precisely this function. For example, years ago, one of the authors encountered an authoritarian and highly moral physician, the husband of a woman who had been admitted to an inpatient service following a serious suicide attempt. He was a successful professional who had little time for psychological issues in general, and social workers in particular. The inpatient facility required very active participation from family members, including attendance at a minimum of three sessions of family therapy and multiple family group therapy each week. When the family therapist, a social worker, initially called to request that the husband come in, he responded by demanding to know her professional credentials and level of experience. When he heard she was a social worker, he said, "I don't need to see a social worker, I have no financial problems." After she carefully explained her role as the family representative of a multidiscipline team, he reluctantly agreed to attend the first assessment session. He left this rather tense session claiming it was "moderately useful," and agreeing to a second appointment. Two days later, he called to cancel this appointment. His voice dripping with hostility, he used the following explanation: "I've been thinking it over, and I've decided all of my problems with my wife are sexual. As a single woman, you couldn't possibly know anything about sex, or *do* you?" This maneuver got him "off the hook" by putting the therapist in a no-win position. If she said she didn't know about sex, he could assert that she couldn't help him. If she, as a single woman, said she did know about sex, he could disqualify her on moral grounds.

It would be easy for any therapist, but particularly an insecure or inexperienced one, to overrespond to this man's hostility and resistance, missing his pain and his difficulty admitting that he did not know, like, or understand what was happening to him in this crisis. It is difficult for most therapists not to become defensive, even when the challenges to the therapist's competence are not serious and hostile attempts to sandbag the therapist but expressions of genuine concern about whether the therapist can be helpful. It is the tendency to respond in kind, to take the challenge personally, to get defensive, that causes normal transient challenges to develop into destructive and pointless power struggles which no one can win.

Challenges to the therapist's competence can actually be provoked by factors other than the therapist's anxiety or the family's attempts to avoid a focus on their problems. They also can be provoked by the therapist's participation in the therapeutic process. The therapist's personal or professional issues may cause him/her to become irrationally or emotionally involved in family systems, and to form involuntary (and perhaps unconscious) alliances with one or more family members. As a result of such unwitting alliances or triangulations involving the therapist, family members may sense that interventions are "out of line" and begin to resist. Most often these resistances can serve as valuable clues to therapists about the timing, accuracy, and appropriateness of their interventions. Challenges only become problems when they create an interaction between the therapist and the family which furthers the cause of resistance.

Challenges to the therapist's competence usually fall into two categories: (1) challenges about personal qualifications; (2) challenges about professional qualifications. Challenges in the personal category tend to be based on ideas that a good therapist must be similar to the family in all basic characteristics (race, class, ethnic background), and/or must have successfully negotiated his/her own marriage and parenthood in order to be able to help others to do so. Challenges in the professional category tend to assume a correlation between therapeutic competence and advanced degrees or past track records with other families. This chapter will discuss some of the major challenges in each of these two categories, offer some general rules for therapist behavior in meeting, avoiding, or using such challenges, and offer some specific suggestions for intervention in challenging situations.

Challenges about personal qualifications: The myth of the perfect therapist, or the pros and cons of life experience

Inexperienced therapists of any age are victims of their sheer lack of experience at doing therapy, but young therapists are also victims of their lack of life experience. In general, the mature therapist with life experience tends to be more likely to have the patience and realism necessary to sort out the possible from the impossible. As years pass, it becomes easier to impart a little wisdom gained from personal encounters with the vicissitudes of intimate relationships.

If all things were equal, perhaps older more experienced therapists with families of their own would be better at helping families with a similar status. But, all things are never equal. That same life experience can be a trap which works against the veteran therapist as strongly as youth and inexperience work against the beginner. While young family therapists may not understand the pain of an ungrateful child, young students with energy, enthusiasm, and determination may do as good a job or even a *better* one than older, more experienced therapists simply because of the optimism and naiveté they bring to their encounters with families. If therapists have been divorced, they are vulnerable to questions about how they can possibly help other couples to stay together. If therapists have children who have problems, as most children do at some point, they are vulnerable to questions of how they can help other parents to deal effectively with their children. Furthermore, everyone knows a few 50-year-old adolescents who are still fighting battles with their aging parents, employers, and society. Therapists engaged in such struggles would be no more sympathetic to a parent's viewpoint than young therapists who have only recently negotiated the emancipation process. Age isn't everything.

While therapy is an art which includes an important human element, therapists are essentially technicians. Being a therapist does not mean that one can live life any better than others can, just as a skilled cancer surgeon has no greater immunity from cancer. All family therapists have grown up and/or live in families with problems of one sort or another. All family therapists have issues with their own parents, spouses, or children which are unresolved and which predispose them to see situations in a distorted way. Rather than feeling inferior for not being perfect, dwelling on inadequacies, or trying to hide them, the task for therapists is to know and accept their own peculiar vulnerabilities. Only in this way can they use their assets and minimize their liabilities. Family therapists, like any other therapists, have few answers. No personal or professional factor guarantees competence. There are advantages and disadvantages to every personal characteristic (be it age, sex, or marital status) and every professional characteristic (be it discipline, style, or years of experience).

Therapist factors are mostly a problem when they cause therapists to be triangulated into the family system. Triangulation happens when a therapist is drawn into an involuntary and sometimes unconscious alliance with one or more members of a family system. The problem can be caused by an over- or underidentification with one member based on the therapist's past familial relationships or current life situation. For example, a young therapist recently presented a family case to her supervisor in which it became obvious that she was overidentified with the wife to the point that she overlooked important features of the family situation. The wife bitterly complained that her husband had affairs while she was left at home tending to the needs of their two children. The therapist totally focused on this young woman, encouraging her to set limits on her husband's behavior and to require him to participate more in their children's care. The therapist also encouraged her to become more independent and assertive. The woman's husband participated very little in the sessions and tended to regard the therapist with suspicion. He finally asked the therapist if she were married. She reluctantly admitted she was recently divorced. "I'm not surprised," the husband commented sarcastically, leaving the rest of the challenge unspoken.

This young woman had become triangulated between husband and wife because of her own current struggle with becoming more assertive and more independent, and because of the history of her husband's infidelity which she believed had destroyed their marriage. She firmly believed that if she had asserted her wishes earlier, her marriage could have been saved, and she had unconsciously projected this notion onto this family's situation. The husband's question and comment totally sandbagged her, that is, she responded with confusion. It was only in the process of supervision/consultation that she was able to understand why her behavior was less than helpful.

When a therapist has become emotionally overinvolved in a family, the issues involved are usually ones of great importance in the therapist's life. These issues are not always conscious but are often readily identifiable if the therapist can take the time and gain the distance to look at them. Unfortunately, this is not always possible to do before the case has been lost. For example, the therapist treating the case of Lilly, the young woman who suffered from uncontrolled vomiting (see Chapter 3), failed to establish herself inside the family boundary primarily because of her overidentification with Lilly's struggle to assert herself in a rigid family system which denied difference and conflict. This therapist later realized that she was vulnerable to triangulation in this particular family because her own struggle as an adolescent had involved a similar attempt to cope with a rigid family system with the same sorts of covert rules against the expression of conflict and difference.

Therapists who are triangulated into alliances with certain family members lose their ability to see the situation with the necessary degree of objectivity. They also lose their ability to intervene freely. A colleague of the authors' is fond of saying that therapists should be able to say something or its exact opposite, based on what they think, not what they feel. If therapists are emotionally involved or triangulated, they will usually be capable of only one kind of response. Family members are right to question the competence of such therapists to treat them until they establish some emotional distance.

The question of professional credentials

The problem of professional credentials stems from the difficulty family members have in evaluating what constitutes a good therapist. Most people assume that the length of time required to obtain a degree is related to the recipient's level of skill. They do not differentiate between training in general and training in family therapy in particular. For this reason psychiatrists have more automatic credibility than social workers or nurses, since being a doctor in our culture has a special meaning and status.

The office walls of physicians and dentists frequently display diplomas from medical or dental school and their certifications by various boards of examination, so that their credentials are quite visible. Most family therapists can't do this since to date there is no examining board in the field of family therapy and probably little agreement as to what constitutes an adequately trained practitioner. Families seeking a competent therapist are presented with a bewildering array of degrees, from the familiar MD, PhD, or MSW, to some degrees even most professionals have never heard of. It's not surprising that families are often confused or skeptical. Some families become conservative and stress that they want "a real doctor," an MD, a psychiatrist. Others are so terrified of being labeled crazy that they request a social worker so that they can say, "this is just family counseling, not therapy." Regardless of how it is expressed, family members often implicitly or explicitly request to be told the professional background and credentials of the therapist. This question usually appears within the first few sessions and represents an attempt by family members to assess how much trust they ought to place in the therapist.

While professional credentials are clearly an asset, they also can be a hazard if the therapist appears to take them too seriously. Some holders of advanced degrees tend to see themselves as beyond the question of competence. They use their degrees to put distance between themselves and families, or even between themselves and their own humanity, stimulating resistance. Young physicians may have particular difficulty in this regard since they are less accustomed to challenges, and may be offended and respond with annoyance or surprised defensiveness that families would presume to question their competence. On the other hand, social workers or nurses often make the opposite error; they underestimate themselves and their training, almost agreeing with families who question their competence. They adopt the mentality of "I'm only a student," or "I only have a master's degree," when approaching families. This further stimulates the family's lack of confidence, and may set up the kind of escalating interaction which ends in the destruction of the therapeutic process.

Students sometimes make the mistake of pretending they are not students, covering up the fact that they meet with a supervisor, fearing that fact will endanger their credibility. Nothing could be further from the truth. Ideally, all family therapy should be practiced in a group, that is, therapists of every level of experience should always have some arrangement to discuss their cases with colleagues or supervisors. Discussing cases or reviewing videotapes can reveal how therapists are becoming caught in family systems before families challenge therapists. Experienced therapists are the first to admit that years of training and a string of degrees are little protection against making the same mistake over and over again. Students should emphasize that although they are the designated therapist, they are part of a team. Input from others, including expert supervisors, will also be brought to bear on the family's problem. By emphasizing the fact that they will be discussing the situation with their supervisors, they can assure families that they will get the benefit of both their own and their supervisors' knowledge.

As was said earlier, challenges to the therapist's professional credentials usually reflect the fact that no matter how sophisticated and knowledgeable family members are in other ways, they have no idea how to
assess the credibility of any therapist, much less a family therapist. It is not
unlike the situation most people are faced with when they must have a car
repaired. They know when their car isn't running right, but they don't
know why. They also don't know how to judge the abilities of someone
who claims to be able to fix it. They can go to recognized dealers or to com-
panies which are well known, but as most people have found out, this does
not guarantee the competence of the mechanic who does the work. They
can rely on the recommendations of friends, but they also know their particular car may need a different kind of mechanic. They need to check
things out for themselves. It may seem oversimplistic to compare the problem of finding a good therapist to that of finding a good mechanic, but the
process is probably very similar. Most people are unsure of what is the
matter with them and what to do about it or they wouldn't be seeking
therapy in the first place. There are a few basic guidelines for therapists to
bear in mind when coping with challenges to their competence.

Basic guidelines

Whether it is called countertransference, getting caught in the family
system, or being triangulated, all family therapists have certain vulnerabilities to certain families at certain times. All therapists become caught up in
family systems repeatedly throughout their careers. They make mistakes
over and over again. More irritatingly, they will often be the same mistakes. All therapists must learn to respect the impact of their own issues
and the strength of the emotional pull of families to draw them into responding irrationally, in ways consistent with their own family or those of
a particular family system. Knowing one's own vulnerabilities prevents, to
some degree, being taken completely by surprise and therefore responding
with confusion when this happens. While it is not always possible to know
what one's vulnerabilities will be in given situations before they occur, if
therapists begin to panic, they should recognize that they are probably
dealing with issues that have particular personal significance. At such
times they should try interventions that will allow some time and distance
to understand what it is all about.

Don't be defensive

Therapists often mistakenly assume that a good family is one which is
immediately and totally compliant. If family members initially question a
therapist's qualifications they view it as a sign that the family may not ac-

cept treatment, rather than as a sign of good judgment. If the therapist can remember that a family's attempts to evaluate the therapist's competence, using whatever criteria they can muster, are a natural, expectable, and healthy phenomenon, it should help the therapist to avoid becoming defensive.

It sometimes helps the therapist avoid being defensive if he/she can focus on the underlying concerns of the family. Most often, the direct question also involves such unspoken questions as "Do you understand us?" "Can you help us?" "Do I have an ally in this painful process?" "Do you really care about my point of view?" "Do you see how hard it is for me to let down my guard, to let someone else be in control?" If the therapist still feels personally attacked after attempting to identify the family's underlying concerns, he/she probably has become triangulated, and the attack has been provoked by therapist error. In such instances, being defensive usually serves only to escalate the situation, and to make it impossible to use the feedback given by the family as the valuable aid to effective therapy.

Be prepared

Therapists may expect and encounter problems with the challenges of families for two reasons: their potential vulnerability because they do not know about a particular experience, or their potential vulnerability because they may know about it only too well. The key factor in handling challenges to the therapist's competence is to be aware of one's own vulnerabilities, and therefore to be prepared to deal with questions about them. It is the defensive reactions of most therapists that exacerbate the doubts of families seeking therapy. An ongoing identification of one's assets and liabilities at any given stage in one's career is important. Family therapists, therefore, should regularly take a long look at themselves in order to identify the areas in which they are most likely to be confronted. As the boy scouts have long known, it helps to be prepared.

In conducting such self-assessments, therapists must consider those characteristics which are likely to be significant for families in general and those characteristics which are likely to be significant for particular families. For instance, if a therapist looks unusually young, this is likely to be an issue for most families and the therapist should be prepared to discuss it with each new case. A therapist's religion, on the other hand, is less likely to be an issue unless he/she is a Protestant seeing an Orthodox Jewish family, or an atheist treating born-again Christians. Since each family brings its own issues, and the issues of therapists will change over time, it's obvious that therapists cannot do one assessment of their characteristics and let it go at that. For instance, dealing with parents who are having trouble agreeing on who should be responsible for which aspects of child care may not be an issue for the newly married therapist. But it may well be a highly charged issue which affects his/her ability to deal with such parents three years later after the therapist has had twins. Preparing for challenges to their competence is an ongoing process for therapists.

Evaluate the context

As with any other type of resistance it is always important to look at the sequence of events in general and the therapist's interventions in particular to understand why a challenge of the therapist has occurred. While early questions may be stimulated by factors unrelated to the therapist's actual behavior, such as the family's fears or stereotypes about therapy, or their preconceptions or misunderstandings about the therapist's role, later challenges are far more likely to be the result of the family's reactions to pressures to change or to therapist error.

Challenges of this sort, therefore, can be clues that a therapist is approaching a highly significant area, that his/her timing is off, that he/she has missed some issue, or is perceived to be in an alliance with one part of a family against another. In such instances, challenges are a favor to the therapist, sending a strong message that he/she must more closely attend to the topic at hand and/or his/her own behavior. It is crucial that the therapist ask himself/herself questions such as the following: Why are they challenging me now? What does this particular challenge mean? What did we do (or what didn't we do) last week that might have provoked these questions?"

Again, it is important to note that sometimes a question is just a question. People get curious, particularly between interviews. More frequently than in individual therapy, families share their therapeutic experience and often discuss the therapist and his/her interventions outside the session. In a sense the therapist becomes part of the family. Therefore, before assuming that all questions are challenges, determine whether in fact a challenge has occurred.

Common challenges to the therapist's competence

Problem 1. "What are your professional qualifications?"

While the principles for dealing with this challenge are the same as those to be used with other challenges, it is important for therapists to remember the confusion in the field as a partial cause for confusion on the part of family members. In responding, the trick is usually to explain how a background in (1) psychiatry; (2) nursing; (3) social work; (4) educational psychology (or any of the other seemingly unrelated fields from which rank-and-file family therapists come) relates to competence in family therapy. Naming one's degree helps, but it doesn't answer all the questions a family may have. Fortunately, many people in other jobs and professions either began by being trained at something other than the job they now do, or learned their jobs from the apprentice system, so they can understand that family therapy is an area of specialization within a wider group of professions and is taught primarily on an apprenticeship basis. Of all possible challenges, this one should cause the least amount of defensiveness in therapists, and should be responded to most directly.

Many therapists have been taught to explore the reasons for behaviors before sharing information, so they evade such questions with the traditional psychiatric cliché "Why do you ask?" Ninety-nine percent of the time therapists can assume that families ask such questions because they are worried about whether or not the therapist can help them. Since many families initially operate as though normal rules of social politeness apply in therapeutic encounters, they tend to back off when therapists answer a question with a question, particularly if there are signs of therapist discomfort.

SUGGESTIONS

Normalize the Challenge and the Family's Concern. It is important, therefore, to communicate to the family that it is okay to ask questions about the therapist's qualifications, and that it is reasonable to have concern about his/her competence to help them. These questions and concerns always exist. If the therapist does not label them as discussable, he/she only demonstrates his/her insecurity and drives the family's concerns underground. If the family notes a defensive response on the part of the therapist, not only will their initial questions remain, but they will probably have additional questions. If the family does not operate by following the rules of social politeness, an evasive or defensive response only gives them a good view of the jugular for which they can aim. Far better to encourage the family to raise questions and to establish a good working climate by giving them permission to do so throughout the course of therapy. The therapist might respond by saying, "I imagine you have some concerns about whether I will be able to help you. Let's talk about that for a minute." If the therapist feels he/she must hear the family's explanation of why they are asking a question about the therapist's qualifications, far better that they should also express a willingness to answer the question. They could say, "I'd be happy to answer that, but first, why do you ask?"

Emphasize the Team Approach. For obvious reasons, students are particularly vulnerable to questions about their professional credentials. Students should always remember that they are part of a team and are being backed up by experienced supervisors and the resources of the agency or institution in which they are serving their internships. This knowledge can give students a sense of competence even when they aren't feeling particularly competent, and can give the families increased confidence in the quality of the overall service that is likely to be provided. This does not necessarily mean deemphasizing the role of student or beginner, but only adding the power of the agency or team working behind the scenes.

Sometimes being a student has its own special advantages in relating to family members. In a recent case, one enterprising student capitalized on his own student role. The presenting patient was a young boy who was having serious troubles in school. His acting-out behavior caused his referral, and that of his family, to the Child Guidance Center. When he was adamant that he did not want to attend, the psychology intern to whom the case was assigned, convinced him to come thusly: "Look, I've been in school all my life. In fact, I'm still in school. I know just about every way possible to have a good time without getting in trouble and I can help you do that, too." The resistant child agreed to come.

Join the Clubs. Sometimes it is possible to avoid the necessity for a long explanation by joining a professional organization such as the American Association for Marriage and Family Therapists or the American Family Therapy Association and telling people you are a member of that organization. Such affiliations are often reassuring to family members who assume that acceptance to such a body relates to competence as a therapist. The authors prefer statements that there are no accrediting boards and that people have to rely on recommendations of people they trust or decide for themselves if they think their therapist is credible and competent. Nevertheless, some kind of certification is reassuring, even when it just says your mechanic went to the Oshkosh School of Auto Mechanics.

Problems 2–7. "You're too: too young/too old; too Black/too White; too male/too female; too married/too single; too childless; too problem free; too different/too much like us."

One of the many objections family members have about therapists is that they are too dissimilar or, more rarely, too similar in some personal aspect. Families always contain individuals of differing ages and sex and, in a pluralistic society, the likelihood is great that a given therapist will not share a similar cultural background or religion with a given family. The problem of differences therefore, is generic to challenges of the therapist's competence. The following is a list of challenges relating to personal characteristics. Since most of the solutions are similar in nature, this problem list will be followed by a list of generic suggestions for interventions. Since some interventions are specific to specific problems, a few suggestions which apply only to specific categories of differences or similarities will also be included.

Problem 2. "You look too young to be a therapist."/"Do you have children of your own?"

In the 1960s, the saying was "Don't trust anyone over 30," but for therapists, the motto is usually the reverse. Those in families with the power to make decisions about the continuation of therapy are usually at least in their 30s and 40s, and may be skeptical of having consultants in their 20s. Youth itself may be the issue. Based on the "you have to be one to treat one" assumption, parents may assume that if therapists haven't successfully negotiated all phases of parenting, they can't help anyone else to do so. In general, it is hard for parents struggling with adolescent children who are physically and sexually active to be upstaged by young therapists enjoying their newly found power. More frequently, however, the issue is really the question of whether the therapist is competent and understanding of their feelings and problems. Often the raising of this question indicates that the parents perceive the therapist already has been insensitive to their needs or is being too supportive of their son or daughter. This may be particularly likely if the therapist is young and/or if the parents and children are locked in an angry struggle with each other. In the latter case, parents assume that if the therapist had ever gone through the problems they are having, he/she would support their position completely and never say anything even remotely friendly to their son or daughter, much less support their offspring's "clearly unreasonable position." The unspoken question is "How could you possibly have had enough experience to cope with a problem as difficult as ours?" In some cases the therapist is only a few years older than the identified patient. Since the parents in such families tend to see the patient as young and incompetent, they may extend this notion to the therapist as well, or worry that the therapist will be likely to side with the patient against them on the basis of their similarity in age.

Problem 3. "You're too old to understand. You remind me of my mother/father/grandmother."

Since grownups are usually too polite to make such observations, and young children think everyone is old, this particular remark is usually made by adolescents or older latency age children. Being over 30 is still considered regretable in this country, so that it is generally considered rude to point to the fact. When children do so, their remarks are often followed by a verbal scuffle in which parents criticize their offspring. This is a tricky situation since, as has been pointed out before, it is a good idea to encourage questions yet it's also a good idea to be initially allied with those people in the family who have the power to determine whether therapy is to continue. The key to a successful intervention, therefore, is to support the parents' protestations about the rudeness of their child while still remaining open to the adolescent or child. This can be accomplished by acknowledging the parents' support with a "Thanks, but . . . " sort of statement and then turning one's attention to the young person with one or more of the suggestions which begin on page 139.

Problem 4. "If you're not successfully married . . . "

This particular challenge to the therapist's competence carries a special twist or two, and should always be responded to thoughtfully. In most societies being single carries special negative connotations. In our own society, until recently, most people who chose not to marry were regarded as sexual and social deviates, and therefore were regarded with suspicion. The responses of most single adults to the question "Are you married?" in everyday conversation have tended to be defensive or explanatory, particularly if the person was near or over 30. In recent years, being single has attained a status of increased legitimacy, but family therapists may still be predisposed to react defensively.

The other twist of this particular challenge for the once-but-no-longer married is the implication that "if you are divorced, how can you expect to be able to help us? . . . " Most families feel that someone who has been married a long time will somehow be better able to repair whatever problems they are having in their marriage. Therapists who have never been married or have been divorced, and feel defensive about this, should recognize this question as a potential trigger of a vulnerable area and, therefore, one which they should think about ahead of time so they can respond thoughtfully rather than emotionally.

Problem 5. "We'd rather work with a male/female therapist."

This particular challenge is almost inevitably present in at least one member of a family or couple coming for therapy, although it is often not stated overtly. Members of couples involved in a struggle with one another may fear that a therapist of the opposite sex will side with their partner against them. On the other hand, some husbands or wives prefer a therapist to be the same sex as their spouse, particularly if they are afraid a therapist may be beguiled by their spouse's charms. Sometimes one spouse is afraid the other won't come, and therefore requests what he/she thinks the other spouse would prefer. For instance, some wives fear that their *macho* husbands will not listen to a female therapist so they request a male. Many adolescents assume that any therapist of the opposite sex is incapable of understanding anything about them, or they are embarrassed about their developing feelings of sexuality and are afraid the opposite sex therapist just might understand their feelings. In any case, gender is an issue, and family members may communicate directly or indirectly that the fact that the therapist just happens to be the sex he/she is makes him/her incapable of treating their particular problem.

In any of the circumstances mentioned above, the preference for the sex of the therapist is often not overtly expressed because of embarrassment over having such feelings as jealousy or fear that the therapist will favor other family members. Therapists should be on the alert for covert expressions of resistance related to the sex of the therapist, particularly those cloaked in overtly humorous remarks about "men/women always sticking together."

In choosing a method for handling this challenge, and in developing a therapeutic style in general, it is important that therapists themselves recognize that there are differences in the ways a male and female therapist can be with a family, particularly if the members of that family have a traditional value orientation. Women would do best to avoid modeling their interventions after the *machismo* of a Walter Kempler or a Salvador Minuchin, particularly if nurturance and subtlety are their forte and the families they are seeing believe that the man should be the head of the house. This may sound and be sexist, but the fact is that families will tolerate different interventions from therapists of different sexes. Beginning therapists of either sex should consider what fits for them (considering their sex and personality), and become comfortable with it. Therapists who are comfortable with a style or an intervention are more likely to make it work for families.

Problem 6. "We want a therapist who is Black/White/Hispanic/ Christian/Jewish/etc."

This is another challenge through which family members try to establish some reason for placing faith in a therapist. Therapists should not be put off by a request for a therapist of another race or religion. It is natural for families to want a therapist whom they believe will intuitively understand them, someone with whom they can identify, someone they think is likely to have similar beliefs, values, and life experiences. It also makes a good deal of sense in terms of accurate diagnosis and treatment. Therapists from a similar background often have many more clues about the problems a family is likely to be encountering and about the ways they will find acceptable for coming to terms with them. Further, they may be more likely to be able to quickly discriminate what kinds of behavior are pathological versus those that are simply variations of particular cultural or subcultural patterns.

For instance, one of the authors was recently called upon to see a couple from Egypt. The wife claimed the husband was crazy and abusive; the husband claimed his wife was unfaithful and lacked respect for him. Both denied the accusations of the other. The therapist found it difficult to differentiate cultural and psychological issues. She knew that in a Muslim marriage, fidelity was extremely important, as was the wife's respect for and submission to her husband. She observed that the wife appeared Westernized and casually comfortable in the setting of her office, while the husband appeared withdrawn and uneasy. As the interview progressed, he seemed to become increasingly controlling of the therapist, correcting her frequently about small details. He also seemed unusually suspicious as he would not sign a document that would only enable the hospital to bill him. In short, he seemed paranoid, the term his wife used in describing his alleged illness. On the other hand, he may simply have been acting as a man brought up in a rural area in Egypt might be expected to act in the office of a female therapist in a Western city, while his wife, raised in a city, was more comfortable. In this case, the therapist might have been more sure of her own abilities to diagnose and help this couple if she had at least been more aware of the beliefs and values of this couple's culture. In most cases the cultural differences will be less dramatic than in this example. More frequently, a White middle-class therapist will be asked to treat a Black or Hispanic family, or a Catholic therapist will be asked to treat a Jewish family.

Problem 7. "You don't understand. You haven't had a child with
    this illness/who attempted suicide/who takes drugs/etc."

At times, parents challenge therapists, saying they have not been through the distress that they are experiencing so that they cannot possibly help. This is particularly likely to occur if the experience is an unusual one that family members have not been able to discuss with other relatives or friends. Parents of the severely mentally or physically ill, for instance, have difficulty accepting direction from therapists who have not gone through the agony of having their child repeatedly attempt suicide, repeatedly require commitment to a mental hospital, or come close to death from a life-endangering physical illness.

GENERIC SUGGESTIONS FOR DEALING WITH PROBLEMS 2–7

The following suggestions are straightforward responses to the relatively straightforward challenges that are inherent in the six problems just described.

Check Out the Family's Concerns. It usually helps to make the family's implicit questions explicit. A therapist should never assume he/she knows what a family is worried about even when the question or challenge seems obvious. He/she must check it out and make the issue explicit. If a family denies that there is any hidden significance to the question, a therapist has at least raised the issue and opened a channel for future discussions of the family's implied concern, should they become more able to express it. A therapist may provide such an opening by saying, "Often people have questions about whether their therapists know what they are doing. If you do have questions, that's okay, just ask." It is important not to ignore subtle hints or half-expressed doubts. When someone asks, "Is that Miss or Mrs.?" the therapist should answer the question, but she should also note that the family may have some concern about her marital status. If a family member asks, "Doesn't your husband mind that you work this late?" the therapist should make a note to check out their fantasies. They may be wondering if she has a husband, if her marriage is good, if she can stand up to her husband, if she is an unfeeling career woman, etc. Since any one of these questions could be contributing to their concerns about whether she can help them, the only way to find out is to ask. Also, asking for the reasons why the therapist's marital status, etc., is being questioned can sometimes provide the therapist with an opportunity to make apparent the illogical nature of the underlying "takes one to treat one" assumption.

The issue, of course, changes depending on who is asking the questions. Parents may be concerned about the competence of a young therapist while the adolescent children may be wondering if an older therapist will take them seriously. Family members may tolerate a particular therapist for some problems that they would not for others. One of our students was well accepted as a therapist by a couple in their 50s as long as the focus of family discussions was on their drug-abusing son. They found the student's youthful curly-headed California look syntonic with their notion of what drug counselors ought to look like. However, as treatment progressed and the focus switched to their marriage, they requested a therapist who was closer to them in years. He respectfully asked them to explain what issues they thought he might not understand. He told them that if he agreed with them after hearing their reasons, he would request they be given an older therapist. By the time they had launched into an explanation of the marital problems he might not understand, and he had made a few helpful interventions, they had forgotten all about their request. The subject never came up again.

Answer the Question. This obvious, straightforward approach to handling this particular form of resistance has often been resolutely avoided by therapists in the helping professions. While avoiding an answer makes sense as a technique in psychodynamically oriented individual therapy where transference is crucial and the patient's fantasies about the therapist are relevant, it is less legitimate in family therapy. The seemingly smug way many therapists have of turning the question back on the client ("Why do you ask?") as a way of keeping the focus on the client's problems rather than the therapist's attributes, also implies that wanting to know the therapist's qualifications is somehow related to a defect in the client's character structure, and has often led to complaints by clients that they can never get a straight answer out of a therapist. Such responses are likely to guarantee that all family members will unite in strengthening their resistance to anything the therapist may subsequently say or do. Giving a direct answer or acknowledging the reality of the situation usually decreases the tension and allows therapists to put into action some of the other suggestions listed below. If they say, "I confess to youth/age; marriage/unmarriage; being male; etc.," in a nondefensive way, the door to a more straightforward discussion of their concerns will be open and they will feel their concerns are being taken seriously.

Explain What People Do and Don't Get from Therapy. One of the reasons people want to have therapists who have experienced a bit of life and have done well with it is not only because this means a therapist is experienced, but because they may have the unrealistic notion that they will inevitably do, value, or be, what the therapist does, values, or is. They believe that if the therapist has a normal family life, then perhaps they will achieve a normal family life. If the therapist is divorced perhaps they will get a divorce. These fantasies reflect unrealistic assumptions about the role of the therapist and the function of therapy. A discussion of the family's ideas or fantasies about the therapist and what these ideas mean to family members can lay the groundwork for an explanation that the family will never become what the therapist is, whether this is desirable or frightening.

For those families who want a therapist who has had their experiences, it may also help to raise the point that there are also potential liabilities in having a therapist who shares too closely the situation they are facing. "Having the same experience sometimes means you have the same blind spots. It may be *helpful* that I'm so different from you." Whenever a family is concerned about differences it may also be reassuring to remind them that by forming a treatment contract they have not given up their power and the right to question and/or reject the views or suggestions of the therapist.

Admit That Differences Might Be a Problem and Appeal for Their Help. This response is particularly useful and effective in early interviews if the resistance is not too serious. People can be caught off guard by candor and an appeal for their help, for example, by a statement such as "No, I've never had a child with a drug problem, in fact, I have no children. Do you think that's a problem?" If such a statement is followed by a request for feedback whenever the family thinks the therapist is missing something important or is not understanding the issues, the family's support and cooperation usually can be enlisted. However, when challenges based on personal differences are very persistent, or when they reoccur later in the therapy, it is important to take them more seriously. While therapists can continue to point out that it is not necessary for them to have experienced everything in order to be helpful, they should examine their own behavior to see if they are unwittingly stimulating resistance.

Ask for a Trial Run. If questions occur early in therapy, the therapist can ask the resistant member(s) to give the therapy a trial period of a certain number of weeks, after which the family and therapist will "reevaluate" together how things are going. This technique can only be used when the complaints of the therapist being too different are relatively straightforward, that is, when they do not constitute a signal that the therapist has been triangulated. Buying time gives the therapist a chance to prove that he/she can be useful despite the liability that is being cited. When a therapist asks for a trial run, the number of sessions requested should be inversely related to the level of family resistance. If a family is very skeptical, the therapist should ask for no more than three or four sessions.

Metacommunicate. When a resistance is designed to sandbag a therapist, it is a good rule to remember to use metacommunication, that is, to comment on what is being said/done by the communication rather than responding to the content of the communication. In the introduction to this chapter, an incident was described in which a resistant physician disqualified an unmarried therapist by implying that she was either inexperienced in sexual matters, or if she wasn't, she was immoral. In that case, the therapist thought a moment and then, rather than responding directly to the challenge, she commented on what the physician had accomplished by his comment. She stated that she was now in a no-win position and couldn't really respond without disqualifying herself in some way. The physician acknowledged the impossibility of the position in which he had placed her by laughing and grudgingly making an appointment. This intervention succeeded because the therapist was able to find a way to avoid the disqualification without becoming defensive herself or putting the physician in a defensive position. While this was by no means the end of his resistant behavior, at least it gave the therapist another session in which to further gain his cooperation and trust.

Express Confusion. In some cases when questions of difference represent triangulation, it may be necessary to play past questions without addressing them directly. This technique involves quasi-addressing the issue but letting the voice trail off so that the family members feel obligated to fill the void by talking, or by posing as so confused that the family members feel obliged to rescue the therapist from his/her confusion. The therapist makes a statement such as "I'm not sure I understand the question . . ." or "I'm a little confused about what's happening. . . ." This would have been an alternative to the metacommunication in the previous example.

The therapist could have ducked the physician's challenge by seeming confused about the point of his question and thus putting pressure on the physician to explain his point of view. This sometimes forces family members who are feeling hostile toward the therapist to explain their objections overtly thus making them more manageable and the situation less tense. It also gives the therapist time to think. To return to the student who was legitimately challenged by a husband because the student was overidentified with his wife, an alternative response would have been to look confused, which she certainly was, and to appeal to the disgusted husband for help in understanding his hostility. He might have gotten involved in an explanation of his side of the argument, at which time the therapist could redirect his comments to help him to talk directly to his wife, removing herself from a destructive triangle. The student could then have had a little time to reassess her own position. The beginning therapist in particular, will quickly appreciate the usefulness of this ploy, particularly when his/her confusion is not all an act.

Use Humor. Humor is often as good a device as honesty to disarm a potentially tense situation. If it is part of a therapist's personality style, and if he/she has read signs in the family's interaction that would lead him/her to believe the family would respond favorably, then there is no reason why a little banter shouldn't be used. The therapist who is being challenged about his/her age might say "I'm only 25, but some days I feel a lot older, does that qualify?" Of course, humorous statements must be followed by an offer to discuss the issue seriously, but the humor can take the sting out of the attack and the tenseness out of the discussion. The use of humor depends upon the personality of the therapist. Persons who do not use humor as a part of their everyday coping skills probably will not use it well in a therapeutic situation. Also, the use of humor demands some skill in knowing when it will be effective and appropriate rather than offensive. Some families would see nothing funny about the remark just noted, while others would enjoy it. A good rule is "When in doubt, don't."

Explore the Issue of Referral. If therapists elicit the objections inherent in challenges to their competence, they must take these objections seriously and listen to them. There are times when a therapist will conclude that it would be advisable to give a particular family to another therapist — either because of the level of the family's resistance, because of the depth of the family's feeling about a particular issue, or because the family is right — for whatever reason he/she as a therapist, will not be able to handle this particular case well. If a therapist, in his/her evaluation thinks that he/she is in over his/her head or that the family's reservations are insurmountable, the case should be referred elsewhere. Referring a case to another therapist does not mean that the therapist is incompetent, but only that the added difficulties presented by a particular combination of family and therapist would make therapy longer, more of a struggle, and more problematic for both. In the case of the recently divorced student therapist discussed earlier in this chapter, it would have been no sign of weakness or incompetence for her to decide not to treat that particular couple at this point in her life. If no other therapist is available, this too can be presented to the family so that a conjoint decision can be made. A therapist may say, "I guess there are some potential liabilities to our working together. Considering these liabilities, I'm willing to try, are you?"

All of the above suggestions are useful in handling most challenges to the therapist's competence which are based on differences or similarities. The following are specific to certain kinds of differences.

YOUTH

Use the Team Approach. Since supervisors are usually enough older than their students to make an obvious difference, it may be useful to actually bring them into an early session. Some clinics have found it useful to have students introduce their supervisors to family members, stressing that while the supervisor will not actually be in the room, he/she will be reviewing the videotapes or discussing the session with the therapist and that as a team both of them will be responsible for the treatment process. This is done in anticipation of the questions family members might have about the youth of most students.

Avoid Challenges by Not Upstaging Parents. Therapists whose youth gives them an obvious affinity for the viewpoints of adolescents and young adults must deemphasize that affinity by not moving too rapidly into the "older and wiser advisor" position with the younger members of the family. This position tends to put the therapist in direct competition with the parents and serves to undermine their authority and competence. In joining with a family or making interventions into their system, the therapist should emphasize the parents' competence to perform their roles.

THE ABSENCE OF YOUTH

Don't Try to Prove You're Hip. When teenagers regard even therapists in their 20s as over the hill and out of touch, it is always a mistake to try to join them on their level. Therapists who are trying to prove they are still hip are usually sending an invitation to be shot down. It is far better for a therapist to accept and admit to his/her own age and identity, but to stress a genuine willingness to hear and respect the adolescent's view. This does not mean the therapist must agree with that view, or that the adolescent will get his/her way, but it does mean that he/she will have a fair hearing. Fairness and sincerity are the keys. Adolescents are experts in detecting insincerity.

Disavow Any Knowledge of the Adolescent Culture. This is a variation of the approach taken with families who actually do come from different cultures. Therapists can engage adolescents by asking them to explain "what's going on nowadays" so that they can better understand the adolescent's position on any issue. Using their ignorance of the adolescent culture, therapists can ask questions which communicate that they are respectful of the adolescent's reality. The resulting discussion can enable therapists to begin to establish a relationship with adolescents.

THE ABSENCE OF MARRIAGE

Admit the Disadvantage but Stress the Assets. A therapist who has not been married usually knows less about the vicissitudes of managing the details of intimate relationships than one who has been married. Since this lack of knowledge is an obvious disadvantage, it's better to admit to it if challenged. Nevertheless, therapists can emphasize that they have been trained to help others to work on their relationships, and that they are very good at doing just that. Further, as was mentioned earlier, the therapist can also emphasize that a marriage of his/her own might result in other liabilities: "I might be a better therapist if I were married. On the other hand, I might just have an ax to grind that would get in the way."

Identify with the Feelings of Despair. The implication of the concern that the therapist is not married may be the feeling that marriage is so difficult that only someone who has managed to survive in one over time could possibly help. Sometimes it's possible for therapists to immediately address the pain and skepticism behind the question. They might state, "It sounds like you're feeling pretty hopeless about change right now." Once couples begin discussing the weighty emotional issues about their own relationship and once they see that the therapist does not wilt at them, they are less concerned about his/her personal status.

GENDER

Bring It Up First. Gender is almost always an issue in family therapy. There is always a difference in either the sex of the therapist and one member of the marital/parental pair, or the sexual orientation of the therapist and that of the couple, or both, as in the case of a heterosexual male therapist treating a lesbian couple. It is often best to state openly that there are differences which could cause problems and therefore the opposite sexed member or members with another orientation ought to be sure the therapist is understanding the issues from his/her point of view. This intervention demonstrates that the therapist is not afraid to discuss the issue but also puts some of the responsibility back onto the family.

Request a Cotherapist or an Opposite-Sex Supervisor. In most cases, objections to a therapist's sex disappear when people have some experience with the therapist and begin to trust that he/she is not blind to their issues because of gender, is not beguiled by their charming spouse, or is intelligent enough for their macho husband to take seriously. However, in some cases, sex does remain an issue which impairs the progress of therapy, either because one family member remains skeptical about the therapist's sex or because the therapist is triangulated because of gender. The latter is much more common. All therapists are subject to intuitively understanding and tending to sympathize with persons of their own sex, or to being unusually hard on persons of their own sex because they aren't living up to their notions of how men or women ought to behave. Since these assumptions and behaviors are difficult for therapists to recognize in themselves, it is frequently useful to have a cotherapist or supervisor who is of the opposite sex and who will occasionally challenge interpretations of what is happening in therapy sessions.

DIFFERENT CULTURE

Take the Time to Explore the Culture. It is not always possible to supply people with therapists who match them on every important sociocultural characteristic such as race, religion, color, and class. Furthermore, such cultural similarities are not always an advantage. As any anthropologist knows, it is far more difficult to study one's own culture than a foreign one, because too many things are taken for granted, and too many blind spots are likely to coincide. The therapist can ask family members to make their cultural values and norms explicit. As the family does this for the therapist, it may also become clear that there are differences between family members in the value and interpretations they place on various aspects of their own culture. Further, their descriptions of their own behaviors and problems can be explored by asking how these behaviors differ from those of other couples or families in their culture. In this way, a therapist's lack of knowledge can be made into an asset. Not only does it force into the open differing expectations and values, but it provides the therapist with an early opportunity to demonstrate that he/she is interested and willing to respect the family's perspective and flexible enough to gauge interventions accordingly.

Check Out Whether Differences with the Dominant Culture Are a Problem. Whether a family is from another country or whether they are members of a subculture within this society, it is possible that their differences with the majority culture cause problems for them. Certainly research suggests that there are negative effects arising from living in an incongruent community. Whether these effects are caused by prejudice, a truncated social network, or whether they reflect some other stress or personality variable, the differences should be explored. The family may not even be aware of the extent of the impact inherent in having to deal with the family–community boundary while absorbing or fighting prejudice and stereotypes. Further, if this cultural group is in a disadvantaged or one-down position, many professionals they have encountered in the past may have failed to respect their behaviors and values. Thus these family members may view professionals as potential adversaries rather than potential helpers. Attending to the issue of how their cultural differences have been an issue in the past may help to communicate respect for the "extra row" they have had to hoe, and may begin to build trust and prevent the development of another negative contact with professionals.

LACK OF SIMILAR PAINFUL EXPERIENCE

Admit You Will Never Know the Depth of Their Distress. None of us can truly experience life as another person does, and many families who come for therapy have had extraordinary experiences. Even experienced family therapists usually have not had the experience of witnessing the progressive personality deterioration of a son or daughter becoming schizophrenic. Unmarried or even married therapists have not had to cope with a suicidal spouse in a manic state or in a severe depression. This does not mean that such a therapist cannot relate to someone who is undergoing this experience. Helping people who have these feelings begins by admitting that the therapist does not know what they have experienced, and listening to their view of what they have been through. This process begins to build an honest therapeutic relationship.

Stress the Experience of Numbers and/or Technical Expertise in Helping Families Learn to Cope. After having admitted that they cannot know all of what a family has been through, and carefully listening to their experiences, a therapist can emphasize that he/she, or the agency, have treated many other families who have had these experiences. Therapists can emphasize that in this process they learned a great deal about what is useful in such crises and have learned how to share this knowledge with families in their situation. The timing of this intervention is all-important. If it is given before families have had an adequate opportunity to communicate what they have experienced, it will be viewed as false reassurance and at best irrelevant. If given after their story has been heard with a sympathetic ear, it may be a welcome relief and may help to establish the therapeutic alliance.

Challenges related to therapist behaviors

An important set of challenges occur both early and later on in treatment which relate more to what therapists have said or done than to their personal or professional qualifications. These challenges are either engendered by triangulation, therapist behaviors which appear inappropriate to family members, or are an inevitable result of the anxieties raised by the therapeutic process.

If therapists are never challenged by families, chances are they are behaving far too supportively and conservatively to produce change in family systems. Family therapists must consistently push family members for different behaviors of one sort or another, whether it be different behaviors toward each other, a different structural organization, or a different level of emotional expression. Therapists must constantly push people to the edge of their tolerance, dancing on the edge of their ambivalence about change without treading so heavily that a severe oppositional response is evoked. When families respond to the therapeutic process with challenges to the therapist's competence, therapists must carefully evaluate whether this resistance is warranted because they have become triangulated or have failed to understand important issues, or whether the resistance is a response to legitimate pressures to change and therefore best confronted as such without backing off or changing direction. The following are examples of these types of challenges.

Problem 8. "You're not fair: You're always on his/her/their side."

Sometimes family members attack the therapists for being unfairly aligned with one or more family members. If therapists are triangulated, this may be a legitimate complaint. Often therapists who are caught in family systems are unaware of their consistent support of one member or one subsystem. This complaint, however, can also be the result of correct interventions and legitimate therapeutic processes. Therapists who are totally "fair" to everyone all the time have probably neutralized themselves altogether. Therapists who are pushing the system toward change will at times strongly support one subsystem or one member to achieve that change, no matter how temporarily "unfair" it may be. It is usually necessary to unbalance a family system to produce a new and more functional balance. Well known as this technique is to family therapists, it often appears arbitrary to family members and results in the charge that the therapist is biased.

SUGGESTIONS

Do a Careful, Honest Appraisal of Your Stand with This Family. Since the challenge is a direct one, and since it is so easy to be caught in a family system, the first avenue for therapists to explore is their own behavior. They must first ask family members for the reasons for the accusations, and what specifically about the therapist's behavior has stimulated these feelings. Next, therapists must take a careful look at these reports, and their own interventions to see if they have been well advised and purposeful or whether they have been emotional reactions to the family system. If they have made an error, therapists should admit it graciously without implying the error is catastrophic. They can say such things as "Maybe I have put a little too much pressure on you, Joe. Let's take a look at that." Most families are pleasantly surprised at this kind of response and do not hold the error against therapists who are flexible and receptive to feedback.

Explain That Therapy, like Life, Isn't Fair. If therapists are firmly esconced inside the family boundary, have an active relationship with all family members, and have determined that they are not overinvolved in the family system, they can teach the family that life isn't fair and that family members must learn to cope with this fact if they are to successfully manage personal relationships. Therapists can use the complaint of unfairness to address the whole issue of reciprocal relationships in hierarchical systems. Adolescents are not the only ones who have the notion that life should be fair and all relationships should be 50–50. Many adults need to be told that there are no 50–50 relationships across the board, that is, relationships may be 50–50 in one area and 60–40 in another. A marital relationship is never totally equal in all areas or it would be a marriage of obsessive clones. A father–son relationship might need to move toward a 50–50 balance as the son matures, but it will never be completely balanced in terms of giving and receiving.

Explain That Effectiveness Is More Important than Fairness. The therapist knows that change does not occur simultaneously in all parts of a family system. While he/she may put more pressure on one member or another at any given time, the therapist has his/her eyes on the overall process, and the ultimate goals of family members. Family members are usually more acutely aware of what is happening at the moment. They may very well forget any previous support the therapist gave them in the face of what appears currently to be an unjust statement or request. A simple reminder that in order to be effective, the therapist must be allowed to determine who is the most ready to change, or who can take pressure at this moment in time, is often sufficient to handle this challenge. For example, Betty and John were referred for marital therapy when the social service department of a hospital found, while doing some routine interviewing after Betty's second miscarriage, that the couple were having serious marital problems. John was described as having had brain surgery for a ruptured aneurysm with the result that he had trouble controlling his impulses. Betty had been putting up with his temper tantrums for four years, but could no longer tolerate them, or the complaints about them from her mother with whom they lived. By the third interview, she had worked herself into a real fury and was close to demanding that John move out of the house. While Betty could see no part she played in John's behavior, the therapist

**To Help Conserve Our
Natural Resources...**

Printed on recycled paper containing a
minimum of 10% post consumer fiber.
The balance is pre-consumer fiber.

BUSINESS REPLY MAIL

FIRST CLASS MAIL   PERMIT NO. 2963-R   WASHINGTON, D.C.

POSTAGE WILL BE PAID BY ADDRESSEE

NATIONAL WILDLIFE FEDERATION

1400 Sixteenth Street, N.W.

Washington, D.C. 20078-6420

could see that Betty systematically agitated John until he lost his temper, a fact which John also realized. He demanded reciprocal change, accusing the therapist of being unfair when she stated that John would have to change first. The therapist acknowledged that the situation looked unfair, but explained to John that Betty was "too angry to change at the moment" and that somebody had to go first. She went on to question John about other situations in which he lost his temper, seizing on the fact that he was able to hold a job, go to school, and drive a car as proof that he did in fact have the strength to hold his temper. John was willing to go along with being the first to change once he understood that he was being defined as "strong" and that it was part of an overall process of reciprocal change.

Problem 9. "We don't seem to be making any progress." ("Are you sure you know what you're doing?")

Impatient with the slowness of change, or discouraged by a particularly regressive incident, family members may turn on the therapist late in the course of treatment and question his/her competence. This challenge is usually not made explicit. In the early stages of therapy such a complaint may take the form of "These sessions seem pretty chaotic," while in the later stages, statements such as "We seem to discuss the same things over and over again" are common. At any stage, a family member may express frustration in the form of "We're not getting anywhere fast!" The implication is that if the therapist were competent, there would be less chaos and confusion, or less repetitive rehashing of old problems, and progress would be swift and obvious.

As has been mentioned repeatedly, these particular challenges must always be evaluated in context to be understood. Why now? If a therapist determines that a family is reacting to something he/she has done, that is, an error in timing, being too aligned with one family member or another, preoccupied with his/her own issues, etc., that behavior should be modified accordingly. For example, if family sessions remain or have become chaotic, the family's complaint is legitimate and a result of therapist error. The therapist must provide the family with a safe, structured arena in which they can discuss issues without anxiety about things getting out of control. The therapist must provide a steady focus so that conflict is resolved rather than avoided and subsequently repeated. In fact, family therapists would do well to listen to the talk-show host Johnny Carson, who, when interviewed by Kenneth Tynan, said, "The only absolute rule is: Never lose control of the show."

The difficulty therapists have in establishing such control and maintaining a steady focus on the issues should not be underestimated. Recently, one of the authors was attempting to make a point about the importance of the therapist taking charge in family sessions to a resident who was also a sports enthusiast. She suggested that his behavior as a family therapist should be like that of the quarterback in a football game, calling the plays to avoid the family's defenses and moving them toward the goal. The resident replied that his sessions with families resembled dodgeball more than football—he never knew where the ball was coming from and he only hoped that if he bobbed and weaved enough, he could stay out of the way and avoid getting hit. Clearly, any complaints a family had about his sessions being chaotic would be a legitimate result of the therapist himself feeling out of control, and his resultant inability to use the sessions to help the family to move toward their goals.

Other therapist errors which can lead families to question competence are therapist overinvolvement and therapist anxiety. The former category includes such items as when the therapist misuses his/her power as a therapist, assuming families necessarily want what the therapist wants for them. The latter category usually involves a situation in which some issue in the family is stirring up anxiety in the therapist and he/she attempts to intervene to increase his/her own comfort rather than to help the family. In a combination of these two therapist errors, a couple in serious marital difficulty was seen by a therapist who had an intense commitment to keeping families together. Although a contract was established which explicitly focused on assessing whether or not the marriage could be preserved, the therapist maintained a hidden agenda to save it. When over time it became increasingly clear that neither partner was committed to the marriage, the therapist increasingly sat on conflict and attempted to smooth things over. She had her own problems with separation and with being responsible for maintaining relationships. She was brought up short when her supervisor observed, "You seem more invested in this marriage than they do."

Not all complaints about the course of therapy, however, are the result of therapist error. Sometimes family members are merely expressing their perceptions about the difficulty of achieving change. Many families secretly wish therapists could surgically remove their problems or wave a magic wand to produce a change. (Many therapists wish they could, too.)

Conversely, covert complaints about the therapist's competence may actually represent family members' anxiety about changes which they already perceive as happening. Response to change is almost always ambivalent.

SUGGESTIONS

Consult with a Supervisor or a Colleague. When implicit complaints about the therapist's competence appear, the therapist may need to change his/her own behavior. To do this, the therapist needs to be able to get some distance from the family in order to be able to develop a sense of perspective. This is best achieved by talking the case over with a supervisor or colleague or, better yet, reviewing videotapes of recent sessions with such a resource person. What may be impossible for therapists to perceive about their own behavior with certain families may be very easy for a third party to see clearly. With the hope of this added perspective, the therapist usually can take the necessary action to impose more control on the sessions or to ease himself/herself out of the overinvolvement. If the problem is that some issue in the family is causing the therapist to become anxious, he/she must decide if the anxiety can be resolved or whether the case must be referred elsewhere. Sometimes awareness of the anxiety-producing issue is enough to begin the process of getting it under control.

Review the Contract with the Family. When family members are expressing the difficulty of achieving change and implying that lack of progress must be the fault of the therapist, it may be useful to review the contract. Given the fits and starts characteristic of any kind of therapy, and the fact that any family member can suddenly become resistant and relapse into previously dysfunctional behaviors, focusing on the contract and what has and hasn't been accomplished lends a sense of perspective to the situation. A review of the contract helps family members to see the positive changes that have occurred, gives them a chance to reevaluate their own goals, and offers a chance for the family to feel a sense of increased control in the therapy. In doing a review, the issues upsetting the family also may become more clear and thus can be resolved directly.

Discuss the Implications of Change. Indirect challenges to the therapist's competence are often a signal that change is beginning to happen. Ambivalence causes members to question the wisdom of all this change and by implication, the wisdom of the therapist. Focusing on the implications of change makes the anxiety overt but leaves the challenge covert. For example, if an irresponsible or provocative adolescent starts acting like a civilized person, parents can be warned that they are about to be deprived of something to complain about. Now they will have to think of something else to talk about besides Johnny's latest act of insolence.

People often need to be reassured that they will retain control over their own lives, and that change will only happen as fast as they can handle it or as fast as they desire it. One depressed young lady seen in the family therapy clinic claimed to desperately desire success in college but continued to fail for reasons that appeared to be related to her dependent relationship with her parents. In family therapy the family made good progress toward the goal of her emancipation, with the patient gradually becoming able to move out of the house and take courses at a local college. Soon after she got her first A at school, she managed to contrive to fail again. She refused to take an exam and gave no excuse to her professor for not doing so. She complained bitterly to the therapist that she obviously needed more help and that perhaps she should try analysis. The therapist responded that she could take as much time as she needed to complete her emancipation, and that she understood that the thought of taking on the responsibilities of adult life was a depressing one. Our patient promptly went home and wrote the make-up exam that her professor, an unusually understanding man, had provided for her.

Problem 10. "You don't care about us."

Families sometimes covertly challenge the therapist's commitment to them, sending unspoken "You don't really care about us" messages, or more accurately, "Prove to me/us that you really care." This form of resistance is particularly common in the middle and end stages of therapy, when the tension level has lowered but difficult issues remain unresolved. These resistances are almost always covert as most families don't want to admit their dependence on the therapist, and overt discussions of the relationship between the therapist and family members is usually not part of a family therapy contract.

Sometimes therapists foster this type of challenge by failing to keep the focus between family members and thereby subtly encouraging them to look to the therapist to meet their needs and solve their problems. This is generally not a good idea in family therapy as families should be learning to meet one another's needs and solve their own problems. In most cases, therapists who receive subtle messages questioning their caring about a family should evaluate whether they have been encouraging too much dependency.

However, in cases in which a family member is severely disturbed, families are often legitmately encouraged to be somewhat dependent on their therapist as part of a long-term treatment plan. The therapist in such cases may insure the continued cooperation of family members by becoming a valuable resource to them in the many crises and trying times involved in coping with chronic illnesses. When therapists use such a long-term approach, they should expect covert messages about the family's feelings of dependency. They should be particularly on the alert for such messages following a vacation, or when, for whatever reason, the therapist has canceled a regular appointment. In some extreme cases, therapists may evoke such a response simply by not being available for a phone call at a time when a family member is feeling particularly distressed.

Challenges to the therapist's commitment may take the form of a verbal comment such as "I left a message for you three hours ago" or they may be acted out in missed appointments or cancellations with weak excuses such as "We didn't think missing one week would hurt." If the therapist does not recognize the resistance, family members may escalate by missing several weeks in a row, may begin voicing more overt challenges, such as complaints about the efficacy of therapy, or they may drift out of treatment altogether.

SUGGESTIONS

Satisfy the Need. Fortunately, this particular challenge is easily handled in most cases. A simple phone call reestablishing contact and concern or an apology for not phoning back earlier is enough to get therapy back on track again. Therapists should remember that most such families neither desire nor will profit by an overt discussion of their dependency on the therapist. Any reasonable expression of caring can modify the challenge sufficiently for therapy to continue.

Escalate to an Authoritarian Position. The ambivalence toward change which is always present can become a major impediment during the later stages of therapy. If a therapist seems uncaring at such a point in time, it may take a bit more than a phone call to communicate that he/she regards the family and the family therapy as important. A therapist may find it helpful to take an authoritarian position regarding the necessity of therapy and the importance of the family keeping their appointments. If a family misses an appointment the therapist can say, "I think it is absolutely crucial that we reschedule this week," and refuse all subsequent attempts by the family to minimize the issue. This usually reassures families that the therapist not only cares about them but that their efforts in therapy are meaningful.

Summary

Direct or indirect challenges to the therapist's competence are as normal and predictable as any other form of resistance to family therapy. They can become destructive to the therapeutic process, however, if the therapist becomes defensive and if an escalating series of interactions between the therapist and one or more family members produces a power struggle. Beginning therapists are most vulnerable to these challenges as they often believe themselves to be incompetent and forget that they have the knowledge and experience of their supervisors and the resources of their agencies and institutions to assist them.

Challenges to the therapist's competence usually arise out of a family's concern as to whether the therapist will be able to help them and mistaken notions of what qualities and qualifications a good therapist should have. Some families rely on advanced degrees while others think that if the therapist is similar to them in race, culture, sex, or a number of other attributes, he/she will automatically be a better therapist for them. Therapists and families alike often make the mistaken assumption that only a therapist who has successfully negotiated all stages of marriage, parenthood, and life is qualified to treat other people's problems.

Challenges to the therapist's competence occur at all stages of therapy although they occur most frequently in the early stages. They may be evoked by therapists who have become unconsciously emotionally overinvolved in a family system or triangulated into the struggles occurring between family members. Other challenges may be the result of therapists imposing their own wishes or goals on families or encouraging the dependency of families when it is not necessary or desirable.

5. Common resistances in ongoing treatment

Habit is habit, and not to be flung out of the window by any man, but coaxed downstairs a step at a time.—Mark Twain

The first few interviews with any family may be the most demanding, but they are also often the most interesting and exciting for the therapist. Every family represents a new challenge, a new therapeutic puzzle to be solved, new individuals to get to know and understand. Since every family is unique, even veteran therapists take keen pleasure in discovering how yet another family operates to cope with their own special realities and problems. When an initial interview goes well, and a reasonable contract is established, both the therapist and the family emerge with a sense of direction and a sense of optimism about the future. Then both must settle down to the processes of ongoing therapy.

Family therapy, like any other treatment, moves in fits and starts. The therapist makes interventions which cause reverberations throughout the family system. As one or another family member begins to change his/her behavior, or the rules of the family system are made explicit or challenged, reactions occur among other family members. These reactions may include positive moves toward the family's goal or regressive moves to restabilize the family system's earlier way of operating. When changes are first encountered, they are likely to be upsetting. As changes are accepted and incorporated, their benefits are more likely to be appreciated. For these reasons, resistances tend to occur in a cyclical rather than continuous fashion. As such, resistances are signals that something is happening in the therapy and their occurence can help therapists to regulate the pace of their interventions.

Resistances in ongoing therapy

In earlier chapters, the therapist was likened to a navigator, and the family members to the captain of a ship. Resistances in ongoing therapy can be defined as all those behaviors which make the ship's journey difficult. Such resistances include all behaviors, feelings, patterns, or styles that operate to prevent change. These resistances may be conscious or unconscious, purposeful or inadvertent, reside in the whole family, in one of its members, or may be distributed throughout the therapeutic system. This chapter will concentrate on resistances within families.

Resistances are conscious and purposeful when one or more family members say, "I don't want to deal with that issue." Resistances are unconscious, yet still purposeful, when family members genuinely believe they want to change, but consistently operate to prevent change from occurring. For example, one woman overtly requested that her husband be more active in disciplining their two adolescent children and then repeatedly found fault with his efforts to do so. She was unaware that she had feelings about giving up her central role in the family and that her criticisms were negative feedback to her husband about his early efforts to change.

Behaviors frequently serve many functions. For our purposes, what is important is not the intent of the behavior, but the function the behavior serves in preventing change. Any behavior, attitude, or property of a family system, whether intended or unconscious, can function as a resistance. For instance, nonstop talkers may not be trying to resist change, but may be simply anxious or operating on the mistaken assumption that the more information they can give the therapist, the more help they will receive. Nevertheless, talking in such instances functions as resistance. Likewise, unrealistic expectations may prevent any movement at all by making it impossible for family members to settle for small but meaningful changes. An attitude of hopelessness may be so demoralizing that family members can put no energy into the work of therapy. In other words, in some instances both idealism and hopelessness operate as resistance.

The style or properties of a family system also may operate as resistances. A family that highly values conformity may be unable to allow conflict to emerge within the therapy sessions, no matter how aware they are that conflict is necessary for the resolution of their difficulties. A family that maintains a rigid focus on the identified patient may be unable to use therapy to change the behaviors of the members that help to maintain the patient's symptom. Family members who consistently blame one another for the problems they have encountered will fail to see their own power to influence the family system. In these examples family patterns operate as resistances to change.

When do resistances occur in ongoing treatment?

Resistances appear both during sessions and between sessions throughout the course of therapy. Of the "during-session" variety, some resistances (e.g., intellectualization, denial, rationalization), are encountered in any type of treatment, yet create special problems when they are manifested in family therapy. Other resistances are peculiar to family therapy (e.g., collusions, family secrets, pseudohostility). All of these resistances can be encountered repeatedly throughout the process of therapy, generally erupting when the family is working on a particularly threatening issue, or when the therapist has made an error in judgment, timing, or has been "caught" by the system.

Many of the resistances encountered in ongoing family treatment are simple repetitions or variations of those encountered in the first session. Others are relevant to the particular phase of therapy or to the particular coping mechanisms of the family. For example, a resistance encountered fairly frequently during the middle stages of therapy, but seldom during early stages, is that of the "pseudocure." While some changes are evident, the magnitude of the change needed to reach the family's goals suddenly appears unacceptable or unattainable to family members. Their solution is to declare themselves cured and happy, or to alter their goals to make it appear that the goals have already been attained.

Between-sessions resistances are often similar to those discussed in Chapters 2 and 3 having to do with attendance or questioning the wisdom of family versus other modes of therapy. For example, when some anxiety-provoking incident has happened during a session or a sensitive issue has been raised, family members may suddenly request individual therapy for a problem family member. Other between-sessions resistances have more to do with failing to follow through on assigned tasks, and undoing whatever changes may have occurred or may be threatening to occur as a result of therapy. All of these behaviors can be viewed as efforts by family members to maintain or reestablish their family status quo.

How does the therapist fit in?

The theory, style, and technique of different therapists will tend to engender different forms and degrees of resistance at varying stages of the therapeutic process. Therapists who begin by making bold interventions into family patterns may encounter enormous and direct resistance in the beginning. Other therapists, such as those with an insight-oriented approach may start more gently, but tend to encounter mounting resistance as serious issues and long-standing disagreements are uncovered.

Depending on their theoretical position, different therapists also will label different behaviors as resistance. How therapists see resistance will relate to their theory of change and the contract they have established with the family. If they believe insight and catharsis to be essential ingredients of change, then the family that uses denial and repression will be seen as resistant even if they follow all other therapeutic directives. The structuralist, on the other hand, seeing no need for insight, will view failure to follow through on assigned tasks as being of greater concern. The gestalt family therapist will view a family as resistant if they do not express their feelings for one another, while the behavioral family therapist will be more concerned with failure to follow through with reinforcement schedules.

If all of these factors are involved, how on earth are therapists who aren't even sure of their theoretical model to know what is resistance and what isn't? After all, the same behavior may or may not be a resistance depending on the person, the family, the therapist, and the stage of therapy. Furthermore, if resistances may be located in the individual, or in the family system, or even move from one person to another and change in their style or presentation, how are therapists to keep up with them? It's fairly easy to recognize massive overt resistances, and it may be all right not to even notice a minor resistance that constitutes nothing more than a passing flirtation wth the status quo. But unless therapists learn to recognize resistance easily, they may only know they are encountering it when they lose a family or begin to feel a case of therapist fatigue. By then it is often too late to save the case. In learning to recognize and deal with resistance in ongoing therapy, the single most important skill therapists can develop is an awareness of patterns and sequences.

The role of patterns and sequences

While every family has thousands of behaviors and issues in its repertoire, every family has characteristic *patterns* of behavior, including characteristic patterns of resistant behavior. Learning to attend to these patterns and sequences of behaviors makes dealing with resistance less complex and more manageable than attempting to attend to each piece of behavior separately. An appreciation of patterns is the key to understanding the function, meaning, and strength of the resistant behaviors and designing strategies to deal with them (Tomm, 1981). All therapists must learn to ask themselves repeatedly, "Why now?" "What just happened that would provoke this behavior, this feeling, this action?" "What does this behavior mean at this point in time?" Every therapist must learn to look to the patterns and sequences of behaviors surrounding any specific behavior that seems to be slowing or preventing the process of change.

In general, in ongoing therapy when some behavior seems to be performing the function of resistance, the first process to examine is the process of therapy itself. Often resistances arise when therapists have missed some important issue, have gotten caught in an alliance with one part of the family, or have asked the family to change too much or too fast. If therapists believe they have provoked resistance, they have two choices: First, they can modify their own behavior in a way that takes this new data into consideration. Small calibrations in therapeutic technique often eradicate the resistance, allowing therapists to move on as before toward established goals. Second, they can focus on the impasse and discuss or use it with the family. This second series of techniques is particularly necessary when therapists have encountered an important, long-term ingrained family pattern, or when they have been slow to pick up a family's signals. At such times families are usually unwilling or unable to forgive and forget without some discussion about what has happened, or some dramatic intervention to modify the struggle. In either case, therapists should first check out their hypothesis that they have caused resistance by making an intervention with the family and observing the response (see also Chapter 4).

This is not to imply that all or even most resistance is provoked by therapists. Rather resistance must be seen as an inevitable part of the interaction between therapist and family. It is also helpful to keep in mind that some resistance is less related to therapy than to the value of the "resistant" behavior in other contexts. For example, a father may have a particularly brusque and demanding style of talking to his teenage children which reduces them to sullen silence. Yet this same style may be very functional at work where he is rewarded for performing an authoritarian role. Unless the therapist understands and acknowledges the influence of occupation on the father's style, he/she may misinterpret the father's reluctance to change this style as simply a resistance to therapy. Once the usefulness of his brusque style in his work has been acknowledged, the father may be more aware of the need for a different style with his teenagers at home, and be more willing to attempt to develop it.

Systems resistance: A case example

The authors have pointed out that resistances are either overt or covert, and that they represent properties of the system, and as such can move from member to member over time, or be active in all members at the same time. An example of a brief therapeutic process will illustrate the myriad ways in which resistance may present itself over time in a single case.

The Trope family was referred for outpatient family therapy after 14-year-old Danny received psychological testing at the University's Psychology Department. He had been referred there for testing by school authorities because of failing grades, truancy, and combative behavior with other children his age and even with teachers. Danny was seen initially with his mother and dad, both in their 40s, and his 21-year-old brother, Josh. His mother, Lyla, and his father, Mike, were quite willing to accept the referral to family therapy despite the fact that they saw Danny as the problem.

The first session

In the first interview, Mike expressed a vague belief that Danny's problems might be related to the whole family, although he wasn't sure how. Meanwhile, his wife sat silently glowering at Danny. The therapist began with the usual questions about the nature of the problem, avoiding everyone's eyes so that the family had to select their own spokesperson. Mike mentioned the testing, indicating that the psychologist claimed the results suggested a family problem, but going on to detail some of the problem behavior exhibited by Danny. The therapist displayed some confusion as to how Danny's behavior could be related to a family problem, and the oldest son, Josh, began the discussion of family issues by explaining that there was a double standard in the house, that Danny was given many more things than he, Josh, had ever had at Danny's age, and that Danny was allowed to do more activities. Mike protested, and the therapist urged them to discuss this disagreement directly with one another. After a few sentences, Lyla interrupted Josh's mild accusation that his father spoiled Danny, stating that it was even worse than Josh was saying. She accused Mike of undermining all the rules she set for Danny. After directly declaring that there was absolutely no parental coalition, Lyla turned to Danny to list a variety of ways in which he took advantage of this situation. Danny remained silent and sullen except for a few grudging monosyllabic answers to the therapist's questions.

The therapist chose not to dwell on Danny's lack of participation but guided the discussion back to the disagreement between his parents regarding Mike's alleged undermining of Lyla's authority. As the open conflict between the parents grew, Josh repeatedly intervened on his mother's side, helping her to make her points. When the anxiety level in the room became intolerable, both Mike and Josh tried to minimize the amount of disagreement. Josh would bring up the problems *he* had had in high school, while Mike, appearing cooperative and reasonable, usually opted out of any responsibility for change by claiming, "I'm doing the best I can." The therapist repeatedly but politely urged Lyla and Mike to continue their discussion, indicating by a lack of response to Josh that while she had earlier favored his contributions, she now wished him to remain silent. The discussion between the parents increased in intensity until Lyla was almost crying. She revealed that she had left home three times the previous year for short periods of time, and intimated she might leave again. Because no reasonable resolution of their conflict seemed immediately feasible, the therapist chose to cool things down to set the stage for assigning a task by making some inquiries unrelated to the relationship between Mike and Lyla. Danny continued to sulk, but did admit that he got along with both parents when he was alone with either one. It was only when all three were together that trouble broke out. The therapist then returned to Mike and Lyla, asking them to negotiate two chores for Danny to accomplish in the following week. Both resisted doing this, allowing Danny to interrupt them with his protests about being assigned any chores and to refocus the entire family on a discussion of who did what with the cat. The therapist, after allowing a polite amount of time to pass, repeatedly returned them to the task at hand. Thirty minutes later they had finally agreed that Danny should take out the garbage every day and move the garbage can to the curb at the end of the week. The therapist, grateful that they had achieved half the requested two chores, quickly assigned Mike to supervise the accomplishment of these tasks, and told Lyla to take a rest from parenting Danny for a week.

DISCUSSION

In this family the early resistances to treatment were minimal and reflected the family's style. Just as the generational boundaries in the family were weak, so were the boundaries between the family and outside influences. This middle-class family, accustomed to ceding power to experts, found it easy to allow the therapist to negotiate the family boundary and assume a position of power. At this point, the only overt resistance to therapy was present in Danny. Typical of many adolescents, and typical of Danny's role in the family, he sulked and refused to participate, expressing everyone's tension and unhappiness. Over the course of the session, it became more and more clear that Danny was a pawn in his parents' power struggle, although a provocative pawn indeed.

Mike consistently tried to minimize Danny's problems and Lyla consistently blamed her husband, neither giving Danny responsibility for his behavior. While Danny was overtly resistant, as the session progressed, it also became clear that Mike was covertly resistant. He used his pseudo-reasonable stance to block any negotiating attempt by either his wife or the therapist. This, of course, provided a therapeutic dilemma for the therapist, for if she had attempted to flush out or challenge Mike's covert resistance, she would seemingly have allied herself with Lyla which might have precipitated more resistance, or even withdrawal from therapy on Mike's part. Josh contributed to the confrontation of family conflict only until the anxiety level exceeded his tolerance. When that occurred he resisted covertly by trying to divert the focus of the discussion to himself.

No one, however, made any attempt to persistently resist the therapist as she redirected the interaction and negotiated the family boundary by slowly taking more and more command of the session. At the point she felt they would accept it, she made the intervention to change the hopeless impasse between the parents. She did not choose to dwell on Lyla's threat to leave as she felt it was too early in the therapeutic process for them to confront the marital issue directly. Instead, she allowed Danny to remain the focus, and assigned a task designed to begin changing the hostile triangular pattern of Lyla directing Danny to do something, Danny resisting, and Mike sabotaging Lyla by either doing the job for Danny or telling him he didn't have to do it. Mike was put in charge of the task and Lyla was told to take a short vacation from disciplining Danny to break this pattern.

The treatment contract actually was concluded almost as an anticlimax to the session. Lyla said she was going to spend the summer working at a resort so that they had only two months to work together. The therapist remarked that they would meet each week until that time to "straighten out this mess with Danny." No mention was made of the obvious marital mess.

The second session

The therapist began the second session by asking about the task. Mike reported that Danny had taken out the garbage every day. Lyla acknowledged that this was true, but then added that she had found one bag which had been dropped in the driveway apparently while Danny was carrying the garbage can to the curb. She related this with a slight note of triumph in her voice. The therapist noted this tone of voice but chose not to comment on it, just as she had not commented directly on Mike's evasiveness during the first session. Mike chose to change the subject. He gravely reported that Danny had been suspended from school for three days because he had bullied another boy into stealing a radio. The therapist interrupted the ensuing bickering between Lyla and Danny and directed Mike to discuss with Lyla what their response to Danny's suspension should be. Mike suggested grounding Danny for a week and Lyla quickly agreed. Danny engaged both of them in a "you'll never be able to make me stay in" argument which the therapist halted in favor of a discussion by Mike and Lyla of just how they would make their punishment stick. Gradually, they took on the job of policing their own discussion, telling Danny to butt out when he interrupted them. During this discussion, both brought up some incidents from the past, revealing that they had once been foster parents of a young orphaned girl, Sherri. Sherri had been a better student than Danny, and the two had competed fiercely in all areas. To break up this competition, they had sent Danny to a private residential school. At the end of their discussion, the therapist reviewed their conclusions about Danny's punishment and the measures they intended to take to insure that Danny stayed in the house for a full week, except for going to school once he was reinstated. During the session, Josh was quiet except for some opening remarks about having spent the week feeding his fish and trying to stay out of the middle of things.

DISCUSSION

Danny's suspension from school was viewed as directly related to the seemingly inconsequential job of taking out the garbage. During the first session, the important issue, and the only one to motivate him to some animated cries of dismay, came when his parents had actually agreed to work together to assign him a chore. He had performed the chore, but had managed to punish his parents for their new alliance and to make a major move to divert them from working together by getting suspended from school. Danny's acting out is one of many types of resistance which occur outside sessions, and is akin to upping the ante at a poker game. Danny's behavior was saying, "Okay, see what you can do with this!" Nevertheless, it was also related to circumstances external to the therapeutic process, that is, the internal workings of his school. The school itself, however, did not appear to be exacerbating Danny's problems to a level which required that the therapist make a direct intervention with the school system, such as calling the principal or making a school visit. (Sometimes other systems such as schools compound the resistance to change and require direct intervention.)

The therapist continued her strategy of promoting a stronger parental coalition by encouraging Lyla and Mike to agree on a response to Danny's expulsion. She did not confront Lyla with the way in which she sought to sabotage the coalition by pointing out that Mike had overlooked a fallen garbage bag, since this would have continued their negative pattern rather than moving on to a more effective one. She urged Mike and Lyla to set consistent limits with Danny, and had them begin by doing so within the session. She regarded a statement by Josh that he had fed his fish and stayed out of the way as his acknowledgment that if his parents were working together, he didn't need to help them parent, but could concentrate on his own concerns.

At this point, the resistance was mostly Danny's and mostly occurred outside the therapy sessions. Mike's covert resistance seemed to diminish after his role as head of the family was reinforced by the therapist putting him in charge of Danny's discipline. Probably for this same reason Lyla's resistance appeared to be on the upswing.

The third session

The therapist received a phone call shortly before the appointed time for the third session. Mike reported that Danny refused to come to the session and asked if he should attempt to physically force him to do so. Since her plan of action at this point was primarily to reinforce the parental coalition, the therapist decided it wasn't worth risking their being defeated in a physical confrontation with Danny over attending the session. She told them to leave both Danny and Josh at home, emphasizing that the father was to point out to Danny that the three of them had decided to go along with his refusal, that is, the parents and the therapist.

The third session began with Mike recounting how Danny had responded to being grounded for a week. After five days of finding that his parents were able to enforce their decision, he had run away. His parents had received a phone call from him 36 hours later, offering to come home if he were granted amnesty. Mike flatly refused and hung up, still not knowing where his son was. Several hours later, Danny showed up.

The therapist expected Lyla to be pleased with Mike's new ability to take a stand, but there was no lessening of her antagonistic tone. After she made several negative remarks on the theme of kids leaving home, the therapist asked what had happened to their foster daughter, Sherri, and why she was no longer a part of the family. The parents related that a struggle had emerged between them after they had accepted Sherri into their home. Mike had felt that his wife was neglecting Danny in favor of Sherri, and in his typical indirect way had dealt with his anger at his wife by getting angry at Sherri. At such times Lyla would defend Sherri, getting into fights with both Mike and Danny over the constant competition between Sherri and Danny. Their initial solution was to send Danny to a private school. After one fairly good year at the school and part of another, Danny heard from Josh that his parents had accepted another foster daughter into their home, supposedly on an emergency and temporary basis, and that the little girl was occupying Danny's room. This was too much for Danny. He ran away from the school and returned home. In the ensuing ruckus, Mike insisted that both foster children be returned to the Child Welfare Department. Again, their solution in a time of trouble had been to send somebody away.

As they related this story, Lyla's whole being became more and more angry. She finally shouted that nothing went on between them anymore, intimating that the marriage was dead. The therapist listened carefully, then stated that they seemed to be struggling over who would have the last word with other things besides Danny, such as how the marriage was to go. She then relabeled Mike's evasive style as "trying to make everybody happy all the time, an impossible task." Mike's way of responding to this intervention was to decide that he must make a choice between his wife and Danny, that obviously he could not make them both happy. His solution? To send Danny away again. The therapist did not oppose his idea nor did she promote it. She simply closed the session, leaving Mike in charge of how to solve the problem of Danny.

DISCUSSION

In this session, while the locus of overt resistance remained with Danny, the locus of covert resistance moved to Lyla. Since her major complaint about her husband was his permissiveness, it was reasonable to expect her to be pleased that Mike had behaved so firmly with Danny. She was far from pleased. She sabotaged any pleasure that either of them could have gained from the accomplishment of a difficult task and diverted other attempts to move forward by sarcastic remarks about her husband's uncaring attitude.

This required that the therapist assess the reasons for the strength of Lyla's resistance to change, a kind of "how angry are you" maneuver. The story of Sherri explained Lyla's deep anger toward Mike and Danny for sending her foster daughters away, and her unresolved sadness about the loss of these children. However, the therapist still felt it was too early in the therapeutic process to focus on the marriage, and Lyla's anger and hurt over the loss of Sherri was clearly still too active for the therapist to risk focusing on it unless she wished to precipitate a crisis. While crises are sometimes necessary to produce change in extremely resistant families, this family was not that resistant. She left the anger and refocused on Mike's evasive attempts to deal with conflictual issues, labeling this as a well-motivated but futile attempt to please everyone. His response was a surprise to the therapist, although given the family's style, it shouldn't have been. Instead of coming to terms with the impossibility of pleasing everyone and the need to unite with his wife to set reasonable limits with Danny, he decided to send him away. The therapist did not oppose the plan openly even though she saw it as poorly thought out and bound to fail. She left the futility of exile as a family coping mechanism for Mike and Lyla to discover on their own.

The fourth session

Lyla opened this session with yet another attack on Mike's competence as a father and husband. Apparently overwhelmed with remorse because of his inquiries into places he could send his son, Mike had tried to make up to Danny by doing something with him. He had taken him out into the garden where they had spent a whole afternoon together planting radishes. When Lyla got home she found they had dug up her prized tulip bulbs in the process, destroying about half of her garden. Understandably, she was livid. She kept bringing up the fact that earlier Mike had offered to let her in on the project, they could have all planted the garden "as a family," saving the tulip bulbs, and presumably the family unity. But, no, he had to go off on his own with Danny, just like always. Mike became increasingly subdued. The therapist quieted Lyla down and then presented her with the notion that it would be hard for her husband to stop acting like a schmuck if she kept calling him one. She seemed surprised at this thought and made a hostile comment to the therapist. Nevertheless, her tone of voice slowly changed a little. The therapist then asked Mike what he had found out about places to send Danny. He reported little luck. He had called several schools and camps for problem children, but Danny did not qualify. The therapist then said she guessed that since they were stuck with the problem, they might as well try to resolve it in therapy. She suggested that the next week, they bring her a list of rules for Danny on which they could agree.

DISCUSSION

The temptation to interpret Mike's digging up Lyla's garden was difficult to resist. Clearly, it was a hostile act, but labeling it as such might have endangered the therapist's tentative relationship with Mike. The therapist had been caught in an unspoken alliance with Lyla ever since the first interview in the sense that in order to stop Mike's evasive behavior she was pushing him to deal with matters more directly which also happened to be Lyla's agenda. To offset this implicit alliance, the therapist finally confronted Lyla with the way in which she contributed to the maintenance of Mike's passive–aggressive behavior. This had the effect of bringing Lyla's covert resistance into the open, as well as increasing Mike's receptivity toward the therapist's suggestion that they jointly create a set of rules.

The fifth and sixth sessions

The fifth session repeated the usual pattern (albeit somewhat muted), of Mike presenting his solution and Lyla minimizing its contribution. The couple had prepared a detailed list of rules and expectations, again starting with the task of taking out the garbage. Although Mike seemed more involved in the process, Lyla's comment about the list was that Danny should have been living under these minimum rules for years. In this interview, their marital tension began to emerge more directly. The therapist labeled their difficulties as serious, focusing on the fact that Lyla's summer job was a kind of miniseparation from which she had not explicitly promised to return. The couple acknowledged the seriousness of their marital problems, but agreed that their first priority was to work together until the summer to get Danny straightened out. They left with instructions to present the list of rules to Danny together when they got home.

A few hours before the next interview, Lyla called the therapist to say that Mike had still not presented the list to Danny and that she was ready to quit therapy. The therapist offered to directly challenge Mike and called him at his job to do so. She discussed the list with Mike who claimed evasively that he had just not gotten around to it. Without hostility or nagging, the therapist emphasized the importance of this move both for the sake of his son and of his marriage. This one issue was the sole focus of the phone call. Mike promised to present the list that very evening and rescheduled the appointment for the following week.

Mike arrived at the sixth session with a big grin on his face, obviously very pleased with himself. He offered a review of the week, inviting Lyla to interrupt him if she did not agree. He then told the following story. After the phone call he and Lyla had presented Danny with the set of rules. Danny took out the garbage for a few days; but on collection day, he failed to move the can to the curb. Mike reminded him several times and then followed him to the basement and ordered him to take out the can. When

Danny refused, Mike went to Danny's room and removed his radio. Danny promptly grabbed a small portable radio which Mike demanded he return. Again, Danny refused, so Mike took it from him forcibly, breaking the antenna. He left Danny in his room after also removing his stereo. A few minutes later, Danny came downstairs to announce that he was calling the police to report his father for stealing and child abuse. Mike refused to allow him to make the phone call whereupon Danny threatened to leave the house. Mike ordered him into his room and shut the door, telling him to stay there. Although Danny kept his parents up half the night singing (apparently to replace the music from his missing radios and stereo), by morning he had become cooperative. Neither the therapist nor Mike and Lyla expected this cooperative behavior to last. Danny would certainly test the rules and limits again. Now, however, both parents knew that Danny could respond to effective limits and that Mike could set them. Mike was pleased with his new ability to take a stand, and even Lyla reluctantly admitted to the therapist that Mike had done well.

This was the last interview before Lyla was to leave for summer at the shore. The therapist summarized the gains of therapy and gave the couple the option of returning for marital sessions in the fall.

DISCUSSION

By the fifth interview, both Mike and Lyla were ready for change to occur, but Lyla's attitude was a skeptical one. She clearly projected the expectation that Mike would fail and the notion that even if he did succeed with this task, it wouldn't be enough. Mike appeared to be at least overtly cooperative and ready to follow through. The therapist allowed a focus on the marital issues both to make them explicit and to label them as possible things to work on in the future, while simultaneously sending the message that no matter how messy the marriage was, she expected the couple to work together to help their son.

When Mike's ambivalence showed itself in passive behaviors between sessions, Lyla was ready and waiting for a hopeless, "I told you so." The therapist was able to get things back on track by intervening directly with Mike. She did not chastise him for his reluctance to change, but she did not back down from the importance of his taking a stand. This head-to-head confrontation was enough to mobilize him into action. In effect, she modeled the firm, fair stance she wanted Mike to take with Danny. The resulting confrontation with Danny was a classic example of a child's response to parents who suddenly begin setting limits and expectations where previously there had been none. While it might seem to have produced a harsh confrontation, a bit of drama is usually necessary to reestablish reasonable generational boundaries. Both Mike and Danny were eventually more comfortable with Mike in charge.

Unfortunately, Lyla's summer job interrupted the therapeutic process. The natural flow of the case would have been to maintain a double focus on Danny and the marital problems until problems with Danny faded, leaving the final sessions to consolidate the marriage. A break in therapy at this point brings with it the risk that the problems with Danny might be sufficiently diminished to decrease the couple's motivation to resolve the marital issues. This is, in fact, what happened. When the therapist called in the fall, Lyla reported that Danny seemed to be doing better in school and was not creating much of a problem at home. She acknowledged that Mike was enforcing the rules they had set for Danny and had largely stopped undermining any discipline she dispensed. She also acknowledged that the marital situation was about the same. However, she stated, since things were so much better, she had decided to use the money she would have spent on therapy to redecorate the house.

Summary

This case illustrates how various degrees of resistance are manifested at different times in different parts of a family system. Danny was always the locus of overt resistance in the system, but resistance appeared to greater or lesser degrees in Mike and Lyla at different points in the therapeutic process. Because this family was only moderately resistant to change, the therapist only confronted the resistance directly on two occasions when she felt the case was in danger of failing. That is, she confronted Lyla's role in maintaining Mike's behavior and she insisted by telephone that Mike present the list of rules to Danny.

This therapist took the view that with this family, resistance would be best handled by avoiding an interpretation of the function of resistant behavior, or even by confronting the way in which resistance operated to perpetuate the family's problems. In fact, it is usually best to avoid such interpretations and confrontations. Confrontations tend to put people in a position with their backs against the wall. Few people change when they are in this position. Having one's back against the wall is a good position from which to fight, but it allows little room to drop back, assess the situation, and pick the most attractive alternative.

Another way to think about it is using the Asian concept of "face." Saving face is very important to everyone, and resistance will always be eased if the therapist finds room for people to change while saving face.

This chapter deals primarily with *diablos conocidos,* that is, the ways in which people resist exchanging their known devils for new ways of relating to each other (see Chapter 1). While these resistant behaviors are described separately for the sake of clarity, always remember that no behavior in a family member is truly separate from the behavior of other members, or from the sequence in which it occurs. The remainder of this chapter will present some of the most common problem situations and some tactical solutions. The suggestions made are geared to get things moving again when they have ground to a halt, or to resolve impasses that otherwise would contribute to therapist fatigue. If any given solution does not work for a particular case, the therapist should reexamine the function of the resistance for the family at this particular point in time.

Common expressions of resistance in ongoing treatment

Problem 1. The too talkative family member

Very often one dominant family member talks nonstop at top volume at times of high anxiety. Other family members sit by and allow the talker to rattle on, to speak for others, and to control the session without being challenged. All attempts by the therapist to involve less active members result in failure as all questions are responded to by "the talker." Such behaviors, of course, may be diagnostic of roles, patterns, and issues in the family system. Before intervening, it is important to determine the role of the person doing the talking, and the function the talking serves in this situation. Beginners tend to equate verbosity in sessions with power, a serious mistake. In a demonstration interview on an inpatient unit, one of the authors interviewed a family which included a teenage girl with anorexia nervosa. The father, a tough marine with a powerful voice and manner, appeared to be the family spokesperson. He talked nonstop. His wife, a nurse, was soft-spoken and rarely said a word unless a question was addressed to her in such a way that she could not defer to her husband. The daughter responded to most questions with "I don't know," or "It really doesn't matter." All three of these family members claimed that the father was the power in the family, and that he made all major decisions. However, nonverbal clues made one wonder about the strength of his power. Often when he spoke, he looked to his wife for her reaction, and if she frowned, he changed his comment midsentence. Late in the interview, when the therapist asked who had decided the daughter should be admitted to the hospital, the father claimed he had, but then casually added that he had really wanted to bring her a year ago, but his wife had said no.

Clearly, in this family, the appearance of male domination was just that, an appearance. The real power in terms of family decision making belonged to the mother. Before jumping to conclusions about the meaning of the behavior of the too talkative member, it is important to assess whether the family has elected this person as a spokesperson, whether this person's talking is allowed in order to provide a smoke screen to cover the anxieties of others, or whether this person is in fact a dominating force in the family. One good clue as to the pervasiveness and everyday presence of this kind of behavior is the ease with which the dominant member accedes to or overrides the comments of other family members, and the degree to which other family members let him/her do so. If other family members spontaneously begin to talk, or do so at the intervention of the therapist, and the talker allows himself/herself to be interrupted, the excessive talking is probably mostly related to the anxiety-producing nature of a family therapy session. If the talker tenaciously continues to dominate the discussion despite attempts at intervention, his/her behavior is probably a pervasive part of the family's patterns of operation. Since a situation-specific behavior will yield far faster and easier than an ingrained behavior, the therapist must make plans for more extended or dramatic interventions.

Whatever the reasons for one person talking excessively, it is important that the therapist not allow any one individual to dominate family sessions on an ongoing basis. If one-member dominance is allowed to continue, the family system continues to operate unchallenged, the therapist fails to establish and maintain himself/herself as in control, and the family may become hopeless of any change ever occurring. If the talker is speaking for others, the first step in changing the system may be to get others to take more responsibility for themselves. If the talker is a smokescreen, the smokescreen must be removed. If a family member is so anxious in therapy sessions that he/she dominates the interviews, the chances are that he/she also behaves this way when things get chaotic in everyday family life. This means it is probably an issue in the family, as well as a behavior the family will be watching as a barometer of how well the therapist can handle their problems.

The reader may recall the psychiatric resident in Chapter 2 who was so overwhelmed by the nonstop talking of a young woman's mother that he asked her to wait in the hall while he interviewed her daughter. Beginning family therapists too often resort to conducting separate individual psychotherapy sessions with each family member rather than confronting the formidable talker in order to gain control of the family session. It is far better to learn a number of methods of dealing with the process of one-member dominance than to develop a pattern of fleeing the scene. Whatever method of dealing with this problem is used, it is important not to "cut down" the too talkative member in such a way that other family members will be afraid to speak, while clearly limiting the process of domination and establishing the therapist's right to control the session.

In this process, it might be helpful to the exasperated therapist to remember that whether people are talking out of anxiety, good intentions (some people really do think that what therapists are after are the facts and that the more facts they can provide, the faster the therapist will be able to solve the mystery of why Johnnie is acting this way, and cure the problem), or actual overt resistance, they usually appreciate and are reassured by limits, structure, and direction. If therapists provide limits and structure and observe the sequences that follow, they will see that resistance almost always diminishes. Here again, an awareness of sequences and patterns can reassure therapists that their interventions were helpful ones.

SUGGESTIONS

Reward and Limit the Speaker. The least confrontive method of dealing with a dominating member is to label this behavior as helpful but as taking too much responsibility for what gets accomplished in a session. The intervention itself might sound something like this: "I appreciate your concern about my understanding what a problem this has been for your family, and it's really important that you have been able to tell me about it. Now, it's also important for me to be able to understand how the other members of your family see this situation." The speaker may yield to this intervention, yet promptly interrupt whoever begins to speak next. It is not at all unusual for it to be necessary for a therapist to intervene in this same manner several times before the dominating member can allow others to have the floor. Nevertheless, consistently interrupting the talker can be done quite graciously, as long as the therapist does not get angry. In our experience, therapists only get angry and impatient if they have let this behavior continue too long and are interrupting out of exasperation rather than therapeutic design. Limits should be set, therefore, as soon as the therapist has decided the behavior does not contribute to the goals of therapy.

Pressure Other Family Members. In a situation in which one member domination is viewed by other family members as negative and controlling, it may help to strategically relabel this behavior based on its positive function for the system. One-member domination may be seen either as overfunctioning on that member's part, or as an effort to make up for the lack of cooperation of other family members. Thus, if the dominant member persists, or if family members are slow to respond once the dominant member is stopped by the therapist, the therapist can accuse other family members of making the talker do all the work. By putting pressure on other family members to participate, the therapist indirectly limits the talker without further stimulating the negative feelings of other family members toward either the talker or the therapist. In essence, this intervention suggests that the talker, however tiresome, is letting the rest of the family off the hook. While this also relabels "helpful" overfunctioning as detrimental to other family members in the long run, it does so in an indirect and nonchallenging way. It redefines the dominance as a property of the system, emphasizes the altruistic intent of negative behavior, and refocuses on the family as a whole.

Employ Nonverbal Techniques. One surefire way of containing an impulsive or compulsive talker is to employ techniques which specifically discourage or forbid talking as a means of expression. Family sculpture and family drawings are just two possibilities in this category. These techniques can equalize the participation of family members, and give added weight to the contributions of those who are usually less articulate. However, the therapist must keep in mind that many compulsive talkers do so out of anxiety and that nonverbal techniques may increase the anxiety level of the talker. Since this may or may not be helpful to the goals of treatment, the therapist must carefully time the use of such techniques, be aware of the probable upsurge of anxiety, and monitor its effect.

Explore the Issue Openly. If the "too talkative member–silent family" pattern is repeated consistently, it may be important to ask the family to describe and react to what happens at home when this sort of thing occurs. Exploration of the myths that exist around the issue may be important, such as each member's fantasy of what would happen if someone interrupted the person doing the talking, or what would be the ramifications for everyone if this person stopped talking. Usually the family will have not considered this option, and the results can sometimes be powerful as family rules are revealed when family members speculate on probable outcomes. For example, the Forbes family was referred to the Family Therapy Clinic because 16-year-old Lisa was clearly depressed. During the first interview, her mother, Diane, talked for everyone. She answered almost all the therapist's questions, regardless of whether they were directed toward any of her three daughters, and particularly if they were directed toward her husband. Since the pattern persisted in later sessions despite attempts to modify it, the therapist pointed out that Diane was doing all the work and went on to ask what might happen if she remained silent. Slowly and nervously, her daughters speculated about what might happen. They concluded that things would probably get very quiet at home. They noted that ever since he had retired, their father had spent more and more time alone in the basement, listening to a portable radio through earphones. Diane's frantic talking seemed to be a desperate effort to cover her husband's depression and the emptiness in the marital relationship, while Lisa's depression seemed both a mirror of her parents' sadness and an expression of her perception of the impossibility of growing up and leaving them to cope with their sadness without her. In fact, the mother and all three daughters were quite concerned about the father. Once this situation had been made explicit, Diane was able to remain quiet while the therapist engaged Lisa's father in a conversation about his retirement. It turned out that he had invested heavily in some equipment which would allow him to continue to support the family by running a small business out of their home. The business had failed to get off the ground and he was feeling useless as a person and as a provider. The family members were able to reassure him of his importance to them, and even to contribute some suggestions about how to get the business going again. All family members brightened considerably, and while this intervention by no means "cured" Lisa's depression, it decreased her mother's anxiety, and got the family therapy moving from a temporary impasse.

Promote Dialogue and Impose "Equal Opportunity" Rules. A good technique to suppress the monologue of the overactive talker is to insist that he/she talk directly to other members of the family. To insure that a dialogue ensues instead of more of the same, the therapist may wish to impose a time limit on each of the speakers. By limiting the comments of all members to 60 seconds, the intervention has an equalizing effect and radically changes the course of the interview. This technique is particularly useful for beginning therapists who are in need of increased control but who have difficulty imposing limits on an ad hoc basis.

A typical therapist intervention of this type might include one of the earlier suggestions, such as labeling the talker as doing all the work, but adding the suggestion that he/she "talk directly to your husband/wife and to your daughters and your son. Ask them to give you a direct answer and be sure not to answer your own question." Since the therapist is dealing with firmly established patterns (if they have persisted beyond initial sessions), he/she should be prepared to repeat these instructions several times before the family members are able to carry them out. Follow-up interventions may be necessary, such as "Did you get an answer to your question? If you didn't, ask it again and wait until he answers," or "Okay, you've said how you feel, don't overwhelm him. Let's hear what he has to say to that."

These techniques also are particularly useful in families in which members chronically blame one another because they tend to stimulate a dialogue rather than allowing one person to report to the therapist about the sins and difficulties of the rest of the family. The therapist may then have the problem of excessive defensiveness on the part of family members, but this is a step forward in terms of changing the family's patterns of interaction.

Problem 2. Chaotic or disruptive children

Unless therapists have spent the first five years of their careers teaching emotionally disturbed children and loving it, there are few things which can unnerve them faster than a roomful of somebody else's loud and unruly children. Even if only one child is disruptive, the entire interview may focus on that child unless the therapist restores order. Many family therapists have had the experience of spending the better part of a therapy hour preventing young children from putting their fingers in electrical outlets or scooping them up just before they knocked videotape cameras through one-way mirrors. It is for this reason that many family therapists ask families to leave infants under the age of 2 or 3 at home after the assessment phase. These children cannot be expected to endure the structure of an interview without presenting a major distraction, or an automatic resistance opportunity which can be stimulated whenever the tension builds. Before expelling children, however, the therapist should always check to make sure parents are not withholding their usual limit-setting behavior so that the therapist can have an unadulterated look at their children's bad behavior, or are operating on the false assumption that the therapist should always be in charge of limit setting in the sessions. In other cases, allowing their children total freedom is seen by parents as a political–philosophical position, more popular in the late 1960s and early 1970s than in the 1980s.

If the parents do see the unruliness as a problem, a common reason they cannot see limits with their children is a fear that their children won't like them. This fear frequently appears in one parent while the other one shrieks at the children in frustration. While this may be a part of a greater marital struggle, some parents seem genuinely afraid their children will reject them if they say, "No." This is a particularly disturbing problem in stepfamilies when the stepparent feels he/she has no mandate or support from the spouse to discipline his/her stepchildren, and that doing so risks rejection by the children and the new mate. This problem can be further exacerbated if the custodial parent refuses to discipline the children adequately out of fear that the children will ask to live with the noncustodial parent. This leaves both parent and stepparent in a position where they are vulnerable to emotional blackmail.

Most frequently, however, the child's or children's disruptiveness functions as a distraction from areas of tension in the family, particularly between the parents. In these cases, the parents often recognize their children's behavior as a problem, but seem powerless to do anything to change it. Their inability to take a stand with their children comes across as ineptness but represents an even more serious problem. On some level, they are afraid to impose order lest the seriousness of their other problems emerge. The function of disruptive children is best assessed by attention to sequences. Do they tend to disrupt when a parent becomes uncomfortable or when tension is building in the marital dyad? If so, the child's behavior is probably symptomatic of parental issues, and constitutes a resistance to dealing with them.

A graduate student in our clinic encountered a classic case of a child's behavior masking serious problems between the parents. Ten-year-old Kevin was referred by his school because of his disruptive behavior in class. His parents had protested to the school that they saw nothing wrong with his behavior, and had accused the school of being prejudiced against their family as they had received some similar complaints about their other children over the years. It was not until Kevin set a fire in their home that they consented to appear for therapy. When Kevin came in with his parents, it was impossible to distinguish his behavior from that of his siblings. All of the children seemed to be completely out of control. Our student tried in vain to establish order. Over the course of many sessions, he urged Kevin's parents to discipline their children, but they merely looked helpless and continued their stream of complaints against the school system. It was not until our student obtained previous records provided by the school that he discovered that both parents had fairly serious drinking problems. Clearly they preferred to maintain the focus on the school system's unfair treatment of their unruly children. It would have been very difficult for the therapist to raise questions about anything other than the children above the din of their shouting.

Frequently a therapist's first inclination is to send the children to the waiting room in order to discuss the situation with their parents in relative peace. This inclination should be stifled for as long as possible if for no other reason than to avoid the eventual retaliation of secretarial staff and colleagues who are trying to get work done. In addition, regardless of the dynamics underlying disruptive behavior, the most important principle is to use that behavior therapeutically. In general, it is best to deal with over-active and disruptive children by getting the parent(s) to do the controlling rather than taking over and doing it for them. In this way, behaviors that have functioned as resistance become opportunities to teach new behaviors to the family and demonstrate to them that they can parent more effectively. Helping parents to deal with the disruptive behavior of their children may not only overcome its use as a resistance, but begin to accomplish an important part of the change necessarily in therapy.

SUGGESTIONS

Educate the Parents about Appropriate Expectations, Rules, etc. In those cases where parents seem to be unaware of appropriate expectations for children, it is a good idea to be quite specific about what rules and expectations children are capable of tolerating. It may be useful to provide some explanation of the difficulties children can experience when they must negotiate school systems which have rules when they have not been exposed to them at home. It may also be necessary to reassure parents that they will not be ruining their children's naturally creative personalities by imposing limits.

A therapist can redefine the reason for application of parental power as "for the good of the child." In doing so, a therapist should point out that no child is developmentally capable of fully determining what is good for him/her and that parents must guide children, particularly when they are in danger of getting out of control. When parents have been ineffective in setting limits, they sometimes resent having to set them almost as much as children resent receiving them. The therapist can neutralize some of the hostility that accompanies this process by stating that it is the job of parents to set limits and the job of children to test them. Setting limits can be defined as part of loving, caring parental behavior. Testing limits can be defined as part of the task of growing up and learning about the world. This explanation is quite useful in stepfamilies as it provides a rationale for either the stepparent or the custodial parent to provide discipline as a part of a loving, caretaking process. If the custodial parent has been discouraging his/her new spouse from behaving like a parent, this will emerge once the rationale has been given, and can be openly dealt with as another issue. Direct education is a first order change intervention and, therefore, should be used first. If it works, it is diagnostic of a simple family problem with few underlying complications. If it doesn't work, it is diagnostic of the fact that there are larger family issues, and it will reveal those issues by highlighting the problems the family raises to circumvent it.

Model and Teach Methods of Control. Nothing works more effectively to demonstrate a point than an immediate experience. For this reason, therapy itself can be used as a practice ground for parents who must become more consistent and effective in limit setting. While it is always better to teach parents to control their children, in some cases therapists may find it necessary to first model methods of getting control over such children. For instance, if parents are unable to set limits on their children, therapists can move in and set the limits themselves, being careful to move out again and turn the control back over to the parent. Modeling methods of control are necessary and effective when children are either verbally or physically abusive to the parents or the therapist, or when their physical activity is destructive. With young children, the therapist can demonstrate to the parent how to use proximity as a behavior control by moving between two difficult children and using touching as a way of cutting down on the number of insults or physical attacks.

The therapist may need to help the family to escalate in their firmness in managing their children. For example, one famous structural family therapist was once observed to actually sit on a 7-year-old boy. This may seem like a radical intervention, but it vividly demonstrated to the boy's parents the degree of firmness needed to reassure their son that they were in control. This boy was the beloved adopted only child of a kindly middle-aged couple who had adopted him after years of trying in vain to have a child of their own. They smothered him with affection, allowing his whims to dictate their lives. From the moment the boy was placed in their home they easily adapted to putting their son's wants and needs ahead of their own. The situation did not become dysfunctional until the boy went to school and encountered the structure of a classroom. His complete inability to sit still and follow directions quickly earned him the label of a disturbed child. The therapist, viewing the boy in the context of his family, quickly ascertained that the boy was more out of control than disturbed in the usual sense of the word. He asked the parents to make the boy clean up the toys he had strewn around the interviewing room. When they proved themselves totally ineffectual the therapist actually sat on the boy until he agreed to clean up the toys, thus dramatically demonstrating to the parents one method of beginning to gain some control over their unruly son. While a therapist wouldn't encourage such a method of limit setting with parents capable of child abuse, for loving, timid parents, it may make a very important point.

Use Behavioral Techniques. When the chaos caused by small children seems to be compounded by parental disorganization, or at least when the chaos is overwhelming to parents, behavior modification techniques are extremely useful. They can provide an efficient way of establishing parental control both within and outside the sessions. Parents can be taught to use token economies, charts with stars or checks, or other reward and punishment systems to establish a sense of structure and predictability for the children and a sense of control for themselves. With a chart prominently displayed on the refrigerator door, it is easy for all to have a sense of whose turn it is to do what, and who is doing well or poorly. Behavioral techniques are often life-savers for single parents who are overloaded with practical and emotional tasks.

Make a Game of Establishing Control. A very useful technique, which to our knowledge was first developed at the Philadelphia Child Guidance Clinic, is to make a game out of establishing parental control. This technique is particularly useful in therapy sessions when there are several disruptive children, when the nature of their disruption is verbal rather than physical, and where the family style tends toward disorganization. The therapist labels an object, such as a hat, ruler, or book the "controller" of the session. Who may speak is determined by who has possession of the object. While the therapist institutes and explains the game, the object is initially turned over to one of the parents. The parent then decides who is to have the object at a given time, thus reinforcing parental authority and control over the children.

Focus on the Function of the Disruption. If a therapist believes a child's disruptive behavior may be serving to distract the family from a more important issue, the therapist, by attending to sequences, should develop a hypothesis about what the overactivity is disrupting. He/she can then bring this process to the family's attention, asking them whether they wish to work on the issue, and if so, to reassure the child that the disruption is not necessary.

A good example of this type of intervention occurred in a session that one of the authors observed several years ago in California at the Family

Therapy Institute in Marin County. A young couple presented with the problem that they couldn't manage their 3-year-old child. Initially, the child was quiet, but as the father became more upset while discussing his relationship with his own father, his 3-year-old son became increasingly disruptive and hyperactive. When the therapist asked the father if he was aware that his son was becoming agitated, the father acknowledged that he was. (It would have been hard to miss since he was literally climbing on his parents.) The therapist then told the father that she thought that the son needed to hear whether or not his father wanted to talk to the therapist about these painful issues. The father turned to the son and said, "Daddy is very upset and Daddy may even cry, but it's okay. I want to do this, it is important to me." The child calmed immediately, and as the session continued, he eventually lay down on the floor between his mother and father and fell asleep. The father and mother continued to discuss highly emotional issues.

Problem 3. The sullen or hostile adolescent

In the interview mentioned earlier in this chapter, Danny presented as a sullen, and for the most part hostile, adolescent. This behavoir can be characteristic of adolescents at any stage of therapy. They are often in a power struggle with their parents and in a period of rebellion toward adults. They don't like talking about their feelings in general, much less with their parents and a strange adult. They arrive at the therapist's office each week coerced and unhappy.

Sometimes an adolescent who has been sullen and silent in the early stages of therapy becomes openly hostile and critical toward the therapist and therapy in general. Increased resistance on the part of an adolescent may often be a sign of changes in the family system that may not even have manifested themselves overtly in family behavior during interviews. For example, when Danny's parents showed the slightest inclination to work together to enforce a punishment for his being expelled from school, Danny became so hostile that he refused to come to therapy at all. Other teenagers may come to therapy, but actively seek to sabotage the sessions. One young lady escalated her mild opening statements that therapy wasn't working and wasn't "enough help" to screams as her family therapist persisted in pursuing the problem the parents had agreeing on issues regarding their children.

Whether they present as sullen or openly hostile, an adolescent's anger can have a profound effect on the family and the therapist. Parents tend to say, "See, we told you, he's hopeless." If the therapist does not intervene effectively, the adolescent gains dominance of the sessions, defeating yet another adult. His/her parents usually conclude that the therapist is no more able to control their rebellious or self-destructive teenager than they are.

Go with the Cooperative Members. In cases where the adolescent is sullen but not openly disruptive, it is often possible to work with cooperative family members until he/she is more willing to participate. The therapist can either ignore the sullen member or can make his/her plan overt, as in "I can see that you're in no mood to talk right now, so I'll work with your parents. If you change your mind, just let us know." The adolescent may be activated when he/she sees that things are moving in a direction seen as unfavorable to himself/herself. This happened in the first interview with Danny when he saw that his parents were going along with the therapist's request that they choose chores for him. He immediately began to lament his loss of freedom, declaring that his social life would be ruined if he had to hang around the house doing chores.

A sullen adolescent may also be drawn into participation when he/she feels the other members of the family are misrepresenting his/her side of an issue. The therapist can promote this by choosing a topic he/she knows is of importance to the adolescent and listening carefully to the parents' point of view. To avoid being seen as too closely allied with the parents, the therapist can express doubts about the parents' statements, such as "It's hard for me to imagine Greg would do that on purpose. Did you ask what his reasons were?" Since Greg's parents are invariably sure they have been more than considerate of his feelings, while Greg sees himself as bullied by his parents, he may be inspired to participate in order to defend his side of the dispute. This technique works equally well when siblings disagree but only those on one side of the argument are willing to talk.

For example, one of the authors was treating a family consisting of a father, stepmother, and four daughters. The second daughter had recently been discharged from the hospital with a diagnosis of anorexia nervosa, and was already rapidly losing weight again. She was sullen, depressed, and refused to speak. Her older sister was openly furious with her parents and the therapist, and for the most part, she wouldn't talk either. However, she eventually was willing to admit that she was also angry with her sister for not eating, and for thus putting herself under restrictions which prevented the two of them from doing all the things they had once loved to do together. As the therapist listened and encouraged these comments, her emaciated sister couldn't tolerate her sister's wrath and made some efforts to defend herself, her first participation in family sessions.

Ask the Adolescent Not to Participate. If the teenager is particularly defiant, the therapist can use a mild paradoxical intervention and ask the silent teenager not to interrupt. This can be done either by labeling the adolescent's silence as having some important stabilizing function in the family, by labeling him/her as not ready to participate, or by labeling the family as not ready to have him/her do so. In any case, the instruction plays into the adolescent's tendency to resist direction and may also play into the competitive nature of many family relationships. For example, two adolescent girls were brought to therapy by their divorced mother, who complained she was having serious difficulties controlling her daughters whom she feared were becoming delinquent. Both daughters refused to speak, saying that their mother had promised them if they came to therapy, they would not have to talk. After some attempts were made to focus on the problems created by this contract the mother had made out of her own sense of powerlessness, the girls were still resistant. The therapist turned to the mother and said, "It's clear that the girls are not yet ready to deal with these problems. They shouldn't talk before they're ready, but you're ready, so let's start with you." In less than a minute, the most resistant daughter began to participate spontaneously, bringing up a more sensitive issue than the one her mother was describing. Soon both daughters were clearly attempting to demonstrate that they were at least as ready to work as their mother.

Frequently adolescents vacillate between sullen silence and hostile denunciations of therapy, the therapist, and life in general. In those cases in which the adolescent is performing a vital tension-deviating function in the family, his/her silence can usually be broken by the instruction not to interrupt and then escalating the tension in the family. Usually the adolescent will be unable to resist interrupting, sometimes with an angry outpouring such as "This isn't going to help. Nothing's going to help. I might as well kill myself." If the therapist is sure the adolescent is making a desperate effort to refocus attention on himself/herself rather than making a genuine threat, he/she can then help the youngster to refocus on the situation at hand and make a more appropriate and useful statement about the situation. One of the authors recently employed this technique with a family in which the oldest daughter had been hospitalized with the diagnosis of borderline personality. Carol created havoc at home and during the sessions by alternating between periods of sullen silence, vicious verbal attacks on her three sisters, and threats to kill herself. Although she claimed she did not wish to participate in family sessions, she consistently attempted to prevent any meaningful interchanges between other family members by refocusing the attention on herself whenever any other topic approached significance. The therapist requested that she not interrupt, reminding her several times by stopping her verbal attacks, and focusing the conversation on the obvious but unacknowledged anger Carol's mother felt for Carol's father. The family's anxiety level rose dramatically, but stabilized when the therapist reassured them that everyone in the family knew about this anger, and that it could be talked about without something terrible happening. For once, Carol joined the discussion in a constructive way, openly admitting her alliance with her mother against her three sisters and their fun-filled but irresponsible father. Gradually her participation in sessions became more constructive, and over time she was eventually able to allow the therapist to move the focus at will without having to create diversions or retreat into sullen silence.

Good Guy, Bad Guy. In cases where two therapists are working with a family, it is possible for one to form an alliance with the parents while the other forms an alliance with the teenager(s). This may begin with the co-therapists taking different sides of the family's battle by talking with each other in front of the family, and then appealing to their various subsystems within the family for support. Having an ally encourages teenagers to talk by assuring that their points will be heard and respected. If they are angry and abusive, it gives the therapist allied with them an opportunity to "suggest" ways in which they can rephrase their thoughts and feelings so that their parents would be more likely to hear them.

For example, in one case a senior therapist was teamed with a student in his 20s. The family consisted of John and Mary, two rather rigid and self-assured pillars of the community, and their three unhappy adolescent children. While the senior therapist was able to sympathize with the agony of the parents over being embarrassed by their children's public displays of disrespect, the younger student drew the children out about their feelings of being overcontrolled and devalued. The student then engaged the senior therapist in a discussion of how she, the senior therapist, had failed to listen to the adolescent's side of the picture. The usual escalation of the adolescents into impotent rage as their parents resolutely became more rigid was replaced by the two therapists reasoning out the situation. Protected by the senior therapist from the threat of their children's rage, the parents were able to hear the other side of the story. The scene concluded with the therapists negotiating a reasonable solution to one of the family's impasses, each turning to their constituency for confirmation of the treaty, after which they shook hands on it and implored their sides to keep the terms of the contract. Later in therapy, the therapists encouraged the two sides to venture to talk with each other directly, at which time each therapist spent most of the time reminding the other to stay out of the middle.

The first three problems we have discussed, the overactive talker, the chaotic family, and the sullen or hostile teenager all have in common the fact that the overt behavior of one or more family members makes it difficult for the therapist to use family sessions to build on the family's strengths to mitigate their difficulties. The next category of problems include more covert properties of the family system in general, or of one member in particular, which function as resistances to therapeutic intervention and change. Families whose style is one of using intellectualization to keep all feelings at bay may not even understand that this style exacerbates or maintains the problems of a specific symptomatic family member. This style may have developed out of a necessity for control of chaos that no longer exists, or may be adaptive in all other parts of member's lives. In such cases, a frontal assault may work, but more than likely, other strategies will be necessary. One can say to the parents of boisterous children, "I can't follow a conversation when everyone's shouting at once." It is more difficult and less effective to say to someone, "I can't get to the point when you rationalize away all the things I see as problematic."

Problem 4. Intellectualization and rationalization

It is only the most chaotic families that do not occasionally use some intellectualization and rationalization to cope with anxiety and maintain control over their environment. These common defense mechanisms only become a problem when they are the only coping mechanisms available to family members and operate to minimize the effect of therapy. Therapists may first notice that their impact is being minimized when what seemed to be a legitimate attempt to identify an issue and engage in problem solving has become a rhetorical debate. They may observe that family members have become invested in the discussion as an end in itself or as a way of justifying their own behaviors rather than reaching a solution to a family problem. If therapists themselves are vulnerable to this style, the problem may progress until they realize they too have been participating in long discussions which do not result in any meaningful change in the family system. If therapists are comfortable with an intellectual approach, or fearful of the magnitude of the underlying feelings in the family, they may inadvertently collude with family members to avoid the stress of change. If therapists find themselves with families that use intellectualization and rationalization, depending on the therapists' philosophy, personality, and skill, they can either adopt an intellectual style of therapy, using it to effect change, or they can short-circuit the intellectualization by using nonverbal, experiential, or paradoxical interventions.

SUGGESTIONS

Use an Intellectual Style of Therapy. An intellectual style of therapy can be very useful as long as the intellectualization is not used as an excuse to avoid making changes or taking action. Family therapy à la Bowen or Boszormenyi-Nagy is a good example of a theory and style of intervention that appeals to therapists and families with such a method of coping with anxiety. Choosing a method of intervention that does not stress the expression of feelings, direct confrontation, or rapid change, may make it easier to join with intellectualizing families, allay their anxieties, and more fully gain their ongoing cooperation. Such models offer family members the opportunity to reenter their families of origin in a way that potentially gives them power and control as opposed to their earlier family experience of feeling overwhelmed, controlled, and impotent. Nevertheless, therapists may encounter some initial resistance to their attempts to use such an approach. For this reason, we will specify a few suggestions to use when initiating this type of family therapy.

1. *Give a logical, intellectual explanation.* When an intellectualizing family presents with a marital problem or a symptomatic child, they may resist the idea of looking at family history or doing a genogram which reveals family patterns and relationships over time. Frequently, they claim not to see the relevance of such information to their current life and their current problems. In such cases, therapists may give logical explanations which show the connections between past family experiences, roles, and patterns, and current problems. They may specifically relate the past to the development of a family member's expectations of a marital partner or a child, or they may speculate about repetitive roles and patterns that are as yet unknown. For instance, when one husband objected to giving family history, claiming he only wanted to evaluate whether or not there was anything left to save in his marriage, the therapist asked, "You mean there was no one else in your family who got a divorce?" He rapidly admitted that his parents had been divorced, but claimed that that had nothing to do with the decision he and his wife were facing. When the therapist asked how old he had been when his parents divorced, and made the connection to his son's current age, he was astounded, interested, and immediately more cooperative.

2. *Move into history as a part of assessment.* If a historical approach is presented as part of gaining complete information about the family in order to choose the correct method of intervention, it has great appeal to the intellectualizing family. They understand the need for facts and plenty of them. As the history is gathered, connections (such as the one mentioned above) can be made and the therapy has begun. Therapy sells itself by its obvious rationality.

Label Feelings as Facts. Rigidly intellectualizing family members may be capable of dealing with feelings if they are legitimized by being labeled as facts. The therapist can adopt the family's intellectual style and explain that while logical explanations are fine, illogical and conflictual feelings are still very real. This worked particularly well with Tim and Barbara, a young couple experiencing marital problems. Both were graduates of an MBA program, had good jobs as junior executives, and were proud of their ability to deal rationally with life's vicissitudes. Nevertheless, Barbara had been referred by her employer because she was experiencing fits of irrational crying on the job. In the course of therapy, the therapist found that the couple had recently moved from Barbara's home city where they had both attended school and where both had unusually good jobs, so that Tim could pursue a particularly attractive job offer. They had, of course, rationally discussed all aspects of the move, including the fact that Barbara might not get as good a job in the new city as Tim had been offered. Still, she agreed to move since she eventually wanted to quit work temporarily to have children, and they both wanted Tim to be in a position to support the family well during that time. Adopting their style, the therapist explained that while Tim and Barbara had probably made a good long-range decision, their short-range problem was that they were ignoring the costs of this decision. Tim and Barbara were surprised to hear about costs, particularly emotional costs, which the therapist delineated item by item: separation from a familiar environment, loss of the support of the extended family, Barbara's loss of prestige in the work setting, her subsequent increased dependency on Tim, and so on down the line. Those feelings of loss had to be faced and resolved rather than ignored, even if the couple did not choose to alter their long-term plans. As homework, the therapist suggested the couple set up a "balance sheet" on which they listed the benefits of their recent move, and the emotional costs of the separation from family and friends, and Barbara's loss of job satisfaction.

Each week the therapist inquired as to the status of the balance sheet, that is, how they stood that week in terms of feeling positively or negatively about their situation. In this way the couple began to deal with their feelings, and to make bargains with each other to ease the situation. For example, Tim insisted Barbara use some of her income to fly to their previous home city at regular intervals so that she would feel less deprived of emotional support. He became more openly supportive, calling her on the job to see how she was feeling. Gradually, they became as competent in negotiating emotional issues as they were in dealing with rational ones. They expanded the number of channels they had available for communication with one another and the world in general. By the end of six sessions, they had learned something about dealing with the less rational but very real side of life, and Barbara's crying spells had disappeared.

Appeal to Authority. Many intellectualizing families find it much easier to tolerate a therapeutic intervention if it is based on some form of authority, either the theraist's, the agency's, or that of an "independent research team." People who intellectualize tend to collect facts to back up their opinions and they are often impressed by hearing such facts used persuasively. A physicist, directly involved in several research projects himself, was referred to the Family Therapy Clinic for marital therapy. He was trying to convince his wife that "open marriage" was the only logical way marriage could survive in this culture. The therapist saw quickly that his wife was totally unable to cope with the idea, but the physicist continued to mount his intellectual argument as to why "open marriages" were superior. The therapist, adapting the intellectual style, quoted a number of follow-up studies on the success of open marriages, noting their poor track record. The physicist accepted these facts and abandoned his intellectual argument, confessing that in reality he felt incapable of monogamy. Soon he and his wife were more appropriately addressing the emotional aspects of his infidelity and her inability to tolerate it.

Use Another Family Member to Comment on the Intellectualizations. In some cases, intellectualization is a total family style, while in others it is only one or two persons who intellectualize. Other members cannot get them to listen to emotional issues or are so awed by their collection of facts or philosophical arguments that they cease to attempt to make their own points. The result is often that other family members become quiet while an intellectualizing member delivers a monologue, or two intellectualizing members engage in a dialogue. In either case there appears to be a collusion to avoid emotional issues. One way to cut through this process is to ask one of the other family members to comment on the ongoing monologue or dialogue.

For example, a history professor and his wife were referred with their disturbed daughter, Dorothy, who had bouts of depression in her teens and currently described herself as having a "hysterical limp." At home, and in many interviews, Dorothy and her father engaged in intellectual dialogues, quite literally about the meaning of life. They referred to German philosophers and Greek poets. The bewildered therapist could barely get a word in. On one occasion when Dorothy and her father started one of these dialogues, the therapist asked Dorothy's mother to comment on the discussion between Dorothy and her father. "Oh, that's been going on since she was little. Always the two of them walking together, talking together, while I follow along behind." The therapist seized on this image of a daughter usurping her mother's position and urged the mother to express some of her feelings about being excluded from the father–daughter interaction. Dorothy's mother's comment allowed the therapist to refocus the interview to begin to modify the powerful father–daughter coalition. In future sessions if Dorothy and her father began their dialogue, the therapist would ask Dorothy's mother to "break it up." Eventually the therapist moved to establish a stronger marital coalition and to encourage Dorothy toward more appropriate peer relationships.

Problem 5. Denial

Denial is another common defense mechanism which can operate as a resistance to therapeutic intervention. It is more difficult to deal with than rationalization and intellectualization because of the tenacity with which people hold onto their beliefs about reality. Some families appear to have logic-tight compartments in their collective "family mind" and if challenged will simply repeat their definitions of reality over and over as if the therapist must be a fool not to see the truth in what is being said.

Denial is particularly common in families that have a strong need to be "the perfect family," or "a really close, loving family." Despite the fact that at least one of their members is exhibiting symptoms of distress severe enough to warrant intervention from the outside, members will cling to the myth that everything in their family is fine, or that everyone except the patient is fine. Families which employ excessive denial also are usually characterized by a high degree of anxiety and frequently regard the therapist as a threat. They resemble the "pseudomutual" families described by Lyman Wynne and his colleagues (1958), or the "consensus-sensitive" families described by David Reiss (Reiss & Sheriff, 1970). Pseudomutuality has been defined as "a family condition in which individuals within the family are predominantly absorbed with fitting together at the expense of differentiating their own personal identities. A family characterized by pseudomutuality views a sense of personal identity as a threat to the whole system of the family" (Wynne, Ryckoff, Day, & Hirsch, 1958, p. 207). As Reiss states, these families seek "an agreed upon rather than a correct interpretation of the environment" (Reiss & Sheriff, 1970, p. 431). While these authors were describing patterns found in schizophrenic families, most clinicians report the same patterns to lesser degrees in many families where individual differences that could potentially cause conflict are denied. Everyone behaves as if it is possible to love and agree with each other all the time. If a family operates as if they believe that differences are destructive, it is very difficult for them to allow the therapist to know about their differences sufficiently to help them to deal with them.

A return to the case of Lilly (see Chapter 2) will demonstrate the concept of extreme denial. Lilly had fits of uncontrollable vomiting for which no organic cause could be found. Her parents, despite obvious differences in temperament, interests, and style, denied any sources of possible conflict in the family. When differences were confronted, they "erased" the implications of their differences by denying that they could have any impact on the family. Fifteen-year-old Lilly faced the impossible task of establishing a separate identity in a family system which could not allow conflict and which erased differences. At one point, the therapist openly suggested that there was an inherent conflict between Lilly's father's demands and her mother's behavior. Desperation overcoming good sense, she asked Lilly to comment on an interaction between her parents which demonstrated their obvious avoidance of conflict. Lilly enthusiastically endorsed the perfection of the parental relationship. In a momentary lapse, her father quite adroitly replied, "If everything's so hunkydory, how come you're throwing up all the time?" He then quickly erased his question and any possibility of

Lilly answering it, with a shrug, and the comment "Well, I guess that's what we're here to find out." But the family really didn't want to find out. Whenever a difference of opinion arose about the family, its members, or anyone's emotions, the family anxiety level rose sufficiently to prompt someone to smooth over the danger with a comment which denied the existence of conflict.

One of the major difficulties beginning therapists have with these families is recognizing what is going on. The family's collusion to maintain a focus on what's right with the family rather than what hurts, or their rigid focus on the symptom, makes it difficult to identify underlying issues. Denial becomes pseudocooperation, as the family maintains the appearance of cooperation with the therapist but remains bewildered about what the therapist could possibly want from them. Gradually, most therapists become inducted into the family's push for symmetry and peace, making it difficult for them to challenge the system and its covert rules. As a result, therapists find themselves conducting "tea parties" with families, in which everyone seems to like one another, but nothing much happens.

SUGGESTIONS

Slow Down. Families with a high degree of denial are usually worried that there really is something unusual or "wrong" with them. Their family boundaries are quite rigid and difficult to negotiate. After many sessions, therapists may still find themselves outside the family boundary and involved in a game of "Problem, Problem, Who's Got a Problem?" Even after therapists have gained some acceptance with family members and have established a treatment contract, they may later inadvertently tread on the family's consensual belief system and find themselves shut out. The danger of therapeutic intervention with these families lies not with simply failing to engage them around their problems in the first or second interview, but rather with frightening them with comments on their family functioning that are too radical at any stage of therapy.

Therefore, therapists receiving signals of increased denial should slow down and even ask the family to slow down as well. They may choose to admit that they themselves had become overly enthusiastic or overly ambitious, stressing the inadvisability of making changes so quickly. Such an intervention may operate directly to reassure the family, or paradoxically, to enhance their sense of control and competence in their ability to move more quickly.

Reinforce the Erased Member. In relatively mild cases of denial, the failure to recognize differences is easy to spot challenge because the family allows some expression of difference but usually fails to acknowledge the expression. For example, a mother may erase her daughter's expression of a difference of opinion by saying, "You don't really meant that," thus failing to acknowledge her daughter's separateness. In many families the denial is expressed by a failure to acknowledge that anything has been said at all; someone changes the subject and the expression of difference gets lost in the conversation. If the members of such families notice that they have been erased or ignored, they usually do not feel competent to challenge other family members about it. Therapists, then, must be vigilant to observe examples of families failing to acknowledge the expression of difference, gently but openly siding with a family member who has been erased, or exhorting him/her to stand up for his/her point of view. They can then instruct family members to continue their discussion with one another, intervening only when denial and erasing interfere. By highlighting small erasures and normalizing differences through such statements as "all families disagree, especially when they love each other a lot because feelings then are so intense," therapists simultaneously can begin to reinforce the separateness of each individual while reinforcing the validity of family loyalties.

If eternal vigilance is the price of freedom, it is also the price of teaching pseudomutual families that differentiation is not necessarily a destructive task. The therapist will have to repeat the intervention described above endlessly before family members take over the function of pointing out erasures to one another.

Use Nonverbal or Experiential Techniques. There are a whole range of experiential techniques which are very useful not only with families in which denial is the predominant coping style but in which rationalization and intellectualization are common. Some experiential techniques, such as family sculpture, dramatize family difficulties and raise the family's anxiety level, while others, such as family drawings allow family members to project potentially anxiety arousing issues onto the task itself. Those families who use an extreme degree of denial are often accessible to the latter sort of techniques, while families in which mild denial is a persistent problem are often responsive to the former type.

For example, Carl and Helen came to family therapy with their two children. Their oldest child, Johnny, was only 5, but had already been labeled by his school as a "peculiar child." He had difficulty getting along with his classmates. Although he was not particularly withdrawn or aggressive, he just didn't seem to fit. The therapist spent several sessions fruitlessly searching for some handle on what the couple might see as problematic either about their son or about the family in general. Everything was fine. The boy's developmental history was fine. His sibling relationship with his little sister was fine. In fact, he had loved her from the moment of her birth and never showed any jealousy and, yes, they considered that normal. The mother–son relationship was fine as was the father–son relationship. The marriage was fine. Even the school was fine. They had no complaints about their child being singled out and would do anything they could to cooperate with the school and the clinic to help their son. Finally, the therapist dug around in the clinic's supply closet until he came up with large sheets of paper and a supply of crayons to use in asking the family to make a family group picture. He asked the family members to jointly draw a picture, either of themselves or of anything they chose. Like Sherlock Holmes the therapist then sat back to observe nonverbal behaviors and the process of interaction to discover clues to family issues and structure. After the artwork was finished, the therapist led a discussion about the resultant picture to see what insights the family might have gained into their own functioning.

In this case, Carl and Helen let Johnny do most of the directing of who was to do what, Carl being particularly hesitant to actively join in. While it was clear that he wasn't used to playing with his children, when he finally sat down on the floor, he seemed to thoroughly enjoy it. The picture the family drew included several typical scenes of their family life. In one scene, the mother and children were bunched together, waving good-bye to the father. In another scene, the mother, father, and daughter were bunched together waving to Johnny who was going off to school. In the final scene, the whole family was bunched together in front of their house, all smiling. The therapist happened to comment that Helen never seemed to be going off anywhere, even to the store. Carl assured the therapist that he did all the shopping even though Helen didn't work. In fact, as the therapist explored this issue, he discovered that Helen never left the house without Carl and even then, only on unusual occasions. From the description of Helen's activities, it appeared she suffered from a mild case of agoraphobia, although she and Carl would not have recognized the name and would have denied the condition had the therapist suggested it. Johnny's strangeness seemed to be a by-product of his mother's self-imposed social isolation. He simply hadn't been exposed to other children or very many social situations outside his own home. The therapist recommended a children's play group which rapidly solved the problem of Johnny's difficulty relating to other children, while the therapist continued meeting with the family. Employing the method of split sessions, he used the first part of each session to teach Carl how to play with his children by using a number of experiential techniques such as puppets or blocks. During the second half of each session, he chatted alone with the parents about their extended families, their neighborhood, and other nonanxiety producing subjects, making suggestions to Helen about joining the PTA and other organizations which might help her son to become less isolated. Helen finally admitted she felt very uncomfortable away from her home, allowing the therapist to talk about the fact that a lot of people felt that way and that special therapists existed who did nothing but treat people who were uncomfortable in certain situations, like being away from home. Eventually, she accepted a referral to an individual behavioral therapist who specialized in phobias, and was greatly helped by a combination of desensitization techniques.

The therapist continued to meet with the family periodically to monitor the inevitable reactions of family members and changes in family functioning as Helen became more functional. Carl, in fact, had a lot of feeling about Helen becoming more independent. Because not all of these feelings were positive, the therapist's continued support was very important. Too often, therapists forget that as the behavior of one member changes (due to individual therapy, medication, or behavior modification), the rest of the family system must make adjustments. Even when the new behavior is a desirable one, care must be taken to help the family to allow change to take place without sabotaging it.

In another case which eventually responded to a nonverbal technique, intellectualization and denial combined to make it almost impossible to gain an inroad into the family's issues. The Stensons were a faculty family suffering from terminal introspection. Both parents were university faculty members who had found intellectualization a successful method of coping with career and personal difficulties. Their family environment was so controlled that their adolescent son had never disagreed with his parents. He was a model child, theirs was a model family. A single but serious act of violence on the son's part brought the family to treatment. The son firebombed the family home. Attempts to deal with this issue in therapy met with consistent denial, intellectualization, and rationalization. The parents claimed they were neither angry nor upset, that they only wished to understand their son's behavior. Even after weeks of therapy, there still was no emotional content to their discussions, and no real willingness to look at family patterns that may have precipitated the incident. For his part, their son Wilfred claimed he had no idea why he had done this destructive act, and stressed that he certainly had no resentment toward his parents.

A nonverbal strategy of intervention helped to break through the family's rigid defenses in order to gain an understanding of the dynamics of the family. The family reluctantly agreed to try "family sculpture," a process in which a family member physically and nonverbally arranges family members according to their emotional roles and relationships. Wilfred sculpted his family in the following manner: He placed his father in one corner, facing the wall, his mother in another corner, facing the wall, and himself in a wastebasket in the center of the room, stretching in both directions. As soon as he had sculpted his family in this manner, his mother burst into tears and the first real exploration of family issues began.

Create a Metaphor. With families employing an extreme degree of denial, the therapist must find a way of introducing the idea or the experience of differentiation without raising the family's anxiety level so high that they cannot assimilate the thought or the experience. Sometimes a metaphor can be a useful vehicle for accomplishing the introduction of the concept. As her first experience in family therapy, a psychiatric resident was assigned the case of Art and Anna, a middle-aged couple, and their two daughters, Kim, 20, and Lisa, 11. The family had been referred by Art's psychiatrist at a VA hospital, who had noticed an exacerbation of Art's chronic anxiety and had inquired about possible causes. Art had told him his older daughter had moved out in a huff after a family fight over her boyfriend.

Art assured the resident he would have no trouble arranging for all family members to attend family therapy, and he was right. All family members were cooperative in attending and participating in family inter-views — as long as the focus of discussion was on Kim's disloyalty in moving out. Art, Anna, and Lisa all agreed that everything had been fine until Kim left home, and that everything would be fine if she returned.

Kim's only defense was that they had been rude to her boyfriend so that she felt compelled to have a place where she could be with him. Session after session, the family danced sadly around this one issue. Art was the only member of the family allowed to express anger, and only at Kim, and only over the issue of her moving out. All the therapist's efforts to broaden the focus failed. She complained to her supervisor that trying to move from Kim's act of disloyalty to the issue of separation and differentiation, was like trying to put a cloud in a box. The focus of family interviews kept slipping through her fingers.

In desperation, she began to focus more and more on Kim's little sister, discussing events at school and in the neighborhood. Lisa talked freely as long as the focus was not on family issues. Every time the resident tried to refocus on the family, even Lisa stopped talking. One day, Lisa announced that she had won the "kindness" prize at her school for the second year in a row. Our resident was smiling to herself, thinking how well trained in "kindness" a child becomes in a family which treats any expression of difference as an act of disloyalty, when it occurred to her that she could use the "kindness" prize as a metaphor for how family members treated each other.

She took a matchbook from her purse and declared it the Kindness Prize. While kindness was certainly a worthy goal, she explained, true kindness did not just occur automatically but had to be negotiated by family members who each presented their own side of an issue. Otherwise, kindness was based on a false sense of what was really going on. From now on, she stated, anyone who agreed with someone else "just to be nice," or who was suspected of not telling their true feelings would be awarded the Kindness Prize. In this way, the idea that inevitable differences could be recognized and handled by negotiation was introduced in a way that made it almost a game. As she repeatedly handed the matchbook to a family member who was covering up feelings, the family members eventually accepted the idea of the Kindness Prize and even began awarding it to each other when they thought a member wasn't reporting true feelings. Metaphors are most useful when, like this one, they arise out of the therapy sessions themselves, that is, from some expression by a family member, but they can also be introduced by the therapist who, over the years, can collect relevant metaphors for various situations.

Use a Minor Paradox and Educate/Teach Them That Conflict Isn't So Bad. Paradoxical interventions are effective but must be used carefully with families with long-term patterns of denial. Once the denial is cracked, changes occur quickly, and not always in the expected direction. As small differences emerge in families that are frightened of conflict, it is particularly important that the therapist maintain control of the sessions so that family members can have these first experiences in a protected climate where they can learn that issues can be resolved without people being hurt irrevocably. They must learn, as Virginia Satir says, that there will be "no dead bodies." In addition to protecting the family from things getting out of control, the therapist can educate them about the process and help them to tolerate temporary discomforts by stressing that things might look worse just before they get better.

Adriane and John had been married for over 20 years when they came for marital therapy. Most of that time, Adriane had been attempting to provoke John to get some sort of reaction out of him. John tolerated just about anything, but a recent extramarital affair on Adriane's part had driven him further underground, into almost complete passivity. Adriane dragged him to therapy saying that she would leave him if he didn't come. Marital sessions rapidly ground to an impasse as John claimed to have no complaints about Adriane now that the affair was over. He insisted on adapting to all of her requests and all of her behaviors. Nevertheless, the air was filled with hostility and both said they knew things were just not right. In this case, the therapist prescribed the symptom, adding the request that John verbalize what he was already doing. She asked John to say to Adriane each morning before leaving for work, "I'm not going to fight with you today," putting into words his nonverbal behavior of 20 years. Adriane for her part, was simply to listen. The next week John announced that he wanted a divorce because the exercise had put him in touch with how angry he was with Adriane. Adriane was shocked and upset. The therapist took control and stated that the open expression of anger was a sign of progress, which would give the marital therapy a focus and something on which to work. She forbade all discussion of divorce for a 6-month period, saying that times would be rough, but a 20-year marriage deserved a 6-month attempt at reconciliation. With this safeguard, both John and Adriane were able to express their frustration, anger, and hurt, and eventually were able to build a new relationship out of one that seemed almost hopeless.

Ask a Third Person to Comment. In some cases, it is beneficial to ask a third member to comment on the interchanges between two other members. A limited version of this technique was described for use with families in which intellectualization and rationalization are rampant (see p. 181). Presumably it is possible for the third member to be less defensive since it is not his/her own relationship which is the focus. As in Selvini Palazzoli and associates' concept of circular questioning (1980), a mother can be asked to comment on how things go between a father and son, or a daughter can be asked to comment on a mother–son relationship, and so on. While some structuralists might fear triangulating the third member, this strategy often offers the therapist information about dyads that the dyads themselves could not give, as well as information about the perceptions and feelings of the speaker. Thus, it can provide an inroad to a system in which denial is prevalent.

Problem 6. The pseudohostile family

Some families spend hour after hour of treatment time engaged in loud and noisy arguments about unimportant issues. From the amount of apparent dissension and hostility, the casual observer might conclude that these families are on the verge of separation or divorce, if not homicide. Those who observe such processes over time usually begin to wonder at the amount of energy that seems to be invested in these fights over what seem to be relatively trivial issues. In fact, these rather obvious superficial and noisy splits serve to cover or mask deeper and more significant ones. Lyman Wynne described this phenomenon at its most extreme in families of schizophrenics (Wynne, 1961), but again, the pattern can be seen to varying degrees in families with a wide variety of problems. It is not always clear whether this "pseudohostility" serves to cover issues about which there would be even more serious disagreement, or whether it serves the function of providing psychological distance when pressures toward intimacy and affection become intolerable. Perhaps both dynamics are relevant at different times in different families. Whatever the reason, families with this style may be viewed as resistant because, unless the therapist can cut through the continuous barrage of meaningless banter, not much can happen to change the patterns of the family system.

Whether one looks on pseudohostility as a fear of intimacy, or a fear of dealing with deeper conflicts, the logical course is to help the family to deal with the underlying issues while the therapist provides a protective context so that the family will not fear being swept away in a wave of togetherness or a wave of murderous rage and subsequent abandonment. The following case example illustrates a "pseudohostile" couple. Jerry and Monica bickered constantly about the division of child-care/household tasks in their marriage. Since they were a dual-career family, Monica felt that Jerry should do as much as she did, whether it was necessary or not. Logical attempts to resolve this issue were rejected, as were any attempts to focus on other issues in the family. Neither Jerry nor Monica was willing to bend 5 percent to create enough good will to work toward a compromise. Nor was either party willing to consider leaving therapy or ending the marriage. The deeper issue for this couple turned out to be a pervasive fear on Monica's part that Jerry did not love her, and a resentment on Jerry's part that Monica had "trapped" him into marriage through an unplanned pregnancy. The problem of their forced marriage had never been discussed since Monica feared and resented what she might hear from Jerry, and Jerry felt his resentment might destroy Monica. The constant bickering about role behaviors was safe, since neither really cared about the reality of who did what. The bickering provided an outlet for their anger and an excuse for the distance between them that they did not know how to bridge.

Patterns of pseudohostility involving two-generational families are also common. For instance, Jim and Beth brought in their three children, claiming they were all impossible to handle. Mike, 18, was drunk all the time, Jason, 13, stole money in school and got caught, and Janie, 11, couldn't get along with either of her siblings. Both parents argued bitterly with first one and then another of their children, and then bickered with each other about which was the most inept parent. Jim accused Beth of spoiling Mike, who he claimed was "her darling," and Beth accused Jim of setting a bad example for all the children by smoking marijuana in front of them. This went on session after session, along with regular reports of chaotic between-sessions fights between Jim and Mike or Jim and Jason. In this particular case, the therapist's efforts to cut through the hostility failed and the family finally achieved a minor amount of peace by sending both Mike and Jason away to school. The therapist warned that this was not a long-term solution and suggested that Jim and Beth come in without the children. They cheerily insisted that they would be fine with only one relatively untroublesome child to worry about. It was not until Jim suddenly demanded a separation that Beth called to state that she realized the difficulties between them could no longer be denied.

It may have occurred to the reader by now that both pseudohostility and pseudomutuality are special kinds of denial. The difference is that, to the uninitiated, the pseudohostile family *appears* to have a great deal of action going on in therapy sessions, while in reality it is a device to maintain the status quo.

Go for the Jugular. If the underlying issue seems clear, or if the therapist has a fairly decent hypothesis about what it might be, it is sometimes possible to cut directly through the barrage of constant attacks. The therapist may simply state, "It seems to me what we're really arguing about here is that you're scared to death this marriage is over." If the therapist is willing to be this blunt whenever pseudohostility occurs, there is at least a 50–50 chance that this technique will work and therapy can proceed to a more productive level. If it doesn't work, little is lost since the family will deny or ignore the therapist's intervention and will simply return to their arguments about irrelevant issues.

Relabel the Hostility as Love. Another way to shut down unproductive pseudohostile communication between family members, particularly between husbands and wives, is to relabel it as their way of making love. The therapist can point out that loving and fighting are essentially the same thing since they are both ways of keeping relationships intense. Such comments as "He wouldn't be so upset over your behavior if he didn't care about you"; "She wouldn't go so far out of her way to agitate you if she didn't love you so much," can be useful. These comments often are sufficient to get people to stop their relentless bickering because they take the steam out of the attack. What good is a really nasty remark if it will lead the other to feel more loved? How much can a nasty remark hurt if it might be a spouse's way of demonstrating caring?

Once the groundwork has been laid, the therapist can relabel the activity as affection whenever sudden outbreaks of pseudohostility occur during the course of treatment, saying something like "There you go making love again. What seems to be happening that could be causing this need to be so affectionate now?" Still later in treatment, family members can be helped to express love and the need for separateness more directly.

Relabel the Hostility as a Distance Maneuver. It is certainly true that some people need more psychological space than others, or have more difficulty tolerating closeness. Family members who feel they should be close to one another, or who feel that they should at least want to be close, sometimes fail to respect their own needs for distance. Psychological distance for such individuals is often achieved through pseudohostility rather than facing the issue that separateness is at times really desirable. Some families can learn to accept that all family members need distance at times, and that it is less painful for all concerned if they can find a way to read the signals of these needs, and find less disturbing ways of achieving or allowing the needed space.

Insist on the "I" Position.   Most pseudohostile families communicate with each other in a steady stream of accusations or disagreements which serve to maintain distance between them and obscure the real issues. Insisting that each person start each sentence with the words "I think" or "I feel" can slow down the interchange of accusations and misinterpretations of each other's motivations, and allow the emergence of individual differentiated positions. The therapist can then underline the importance of maintaining these differentiated positions by simultaneously putting great emphasis on the emerging issue and their emerging strength and ability to handle it more directly. A word of caution when using this intervention. Many family members will obey the letter of this law while ignoring its intent. They immediately switch to "I think *you . . .* " and continue the attack. It is useful to warn them ahead of time that this will not accomplish anything, should be avoided, and will be interrupted by the therapist. For this technique to work, the therapist must interrupt repeatedly, and be comfortable in the role of a "nag." Often these families will fight against assuming responsibility for their own statements. When they finally do, the sessions will become more quiet and more intense as family members try to figure out how to talk to each other in such an unfamiliar manner.

Establish a No Escalation Clause.   A common pattern in pseudohostile families (and in families that play the blame game) is for one member to attack another who, in turn, immediately escalates the level of the attack and raises the volume. This is then either reciprocated by the first member or, more frequently, a third member joins in on either side or opposing them both, escalating the conflict even further. For example, June, 17, was hospitalized because she attacked her mother with a knife. When family therapy was instituted, a typical family interview would begin by June accusing her younger sister Cheryl of some "crime" such as not taking her turn at doing the dishes; Cheryl would then raise her voice, defending herself, and accusing June of taking her radio. The two sisters would then bicker for several minutes until their mother would begin shouting at them about how impossible they both were.

Getting at or resolving the underlying issues and feelings is impossible when this sort of scenario is operating at top volume. To interrupt the circle, therapists can impose a "no escalation clause," that is, they can get all members of the family to agree at the beginning of a session that no one will escalate conflict when it occurs. Therapists then must police the session, stopping all incipient fights before they develop, and monitoring the anxiety level so that family members are not frightened by what happens when no one is yelling. By monitoring the family discussions closely, therapists then are able to enforce their rules that each issue raised be resolved before another can be addressed.

Problem 7. The blame game: A terminal exercise in establishing
   linear causality

The family playing the blame game presents somewhat similarly to
the pseudohostile family. They differ in that the ostensible purpose of the
relentless bickering is not only to obscure difficulties with intimacy, or to
cover deeper underlying issues, but to establish who is to blame for the
family's problems. Etiology is everything. The family acts as if all family
members truly believed that if they could establish "who started it," the
problem would no longer be a problem, or at least only one person would
then have to deal with the problem and the others would be "off the hook."
These families or couples can become stuck in a repetitive interactional
process which centers on who has hurt whom the most over the years of the
marriage and family life cycle. This self-defeating pattern can seem impossible to break. Each person refocuses every communication on the
issue of gaining points, as if there were an imaginary scoreboard in the sky
where the culprit's damning score would someday be revealed at last. The
implication of the blaming is always "If it weren't for *you,* we wouldn't be
in this mess," and by extention, "This mess will only get better when *you*
change *your* behavior or attitude."

The blame game tends to occur mostly between couples, although
adolescents and their parents can be seen to be squared off against each
other in this manner. Whether it is between spouses or between generations, the parties involved tend to trade a continuous stream of accusations. For example, John and Judy, a young couple in their late 20s, presented with severe marital problems. They had married right out of college
where they had experienced an idyllic relationship. Now, eight years later,
both were considering divorce. John attempted to explain philosophically
to the therapist what he thought was happening to the marriage. Judy lost
patience with him and interrupted to say the problem was that John was
totally insensitive to her needs and went on to illustrate an example of his
lack of consideration. John countered with an example of her bitchiness,
clearly enough to inspire the so-called lack of sensitivity even in a saint.
The battle was on. Judy retaliated with one of those "how about the time in
Cincinnati when you . . . " gambits, while John first threw up his hands to
indicate that she was impossible and not worth answering, and then, as
soon as she paused for breath, plunged in with the real killer, "but you're
always on the phone with your mother!" This interaction between them
emerged throughout the course of therapy whenever they hit sensitive
issues such as money, his father, her mother, his need for distance, or her
temper. As is characteristic of effective interventions with families that
play the blame game, the interventions suggested below will probably have
to be repeated many times during the course of therapy.

SUGGESTIONS

Suggest That Establishing Blame Won't Help. This simple common-sense intervention is often overlooked in favor of flashier responses, but it works in a good percentage of cases in which the pattern is of relatively short duration. Most people know that blaming each other isn't going to help, but they are caught in a struggle they don't understand. They feel it's the only way they know of to explain the mess they are in. They feel hopeless about change but believe that establishing blame will at least make something perfectly clear. They need and can respond to someone in authority who gives them a face-saving way to stop a pointless process. The therapist can simply and repeatedly say, "It really won't help to decide who started it, the question is what are we going to do to make it better now?"

Use Logic to Establish What Would Happen if Blame Were Proven. If the first suggestion doesn't work, the therapist can suggest that the family talk together about what they think would happen if they finally could establish who was to blame, or at least, who was mostly to blame for the family's problems. How would that help the situations? Again, the therapist will have to be pretty persistent and repetitive with these questions. Most people have one or two easy responses, such as "Everything would be okay if he only admitted he was wrong." The therapist must pursue such comments with others like, "How could that make it okay?" Most people eventually are forced to admit that establishing causality would not be useful, or worse, might mean the family should take some action they wish to avoid, such as the dissolution of the family as a unit.

Use a Metaphor. Metaphors are handy for saving face in that they often provide a vehicle for people to change without having to admit that they've been mistaken, or that their ways of coping haven't worked. In this case, a metaphor such as "the great scoreboard in the sky," used with a touch of humor, can sometimes help family members to give up this kind of preoccupation with blame. Sometimes a stronger metaphor is needed. For instance, the point could be made that if international misunderstandings caused Russia and United States to begin a war which resulted in a worldwide nuclear holocaust, prolonged debates might eventually determine who started it or who was to blame, but in the meantime, most of us would be dead. The therapist might even add, "The same could be true of your family relationships. Even if we could find the origin of the problem, it might be too late to do any good." Granted this is a pretty extreme example, but sometimes the shock value of such dramatic metaphors is very useful when people are so entrenched in the battle they have lost sight of the cost.

Redirect the Competitive Energy. The blame game is usually carried on with a great deal of competitive spirit. It takes spirit and endurance to play, and therefore the persons engaged in doing so are often quite capable of producing change quickly if therapists can divert their competitive energy from a search for causality to a more positive arena. Using their best judgment of which partner is more capable of change at the moment by assessing which partner has displayed less telltale rigidity or defensiveness, therapists can label that person as "the strongest," or "the most able to change," or the "most ready," whatever seems reasonable to the situation. Therapists can then require that person to be the initiator of change in the family, and make a specific suggestion as to what the person should do to initiate change. In doing so, the therapist readily admits to the family that this may not be fair, but that it will be effective. For example, in the case of John and Judy, John had displayed signs of rigidity by failing to alter his behavior even slightly in response to the therapist's comments over a period of several weeks. Furthermore, certain historical facts emerged which indicated that he was the more vulnerable partner. The therapist suggested to Judy that she would have to change before John could do so, and that what she had to do was to eradicate any trace of the "arrogance" in her voice which so annoyed John. The therapist had noted that John tensed whenever Judy used a certain tone. She labeled it "arrogant," which seemed preferable to the more accurately descriptive "martyred." This accomplished not only a change in the couple's interactions but an effort on John's part to respond with a reciprocal move of his own, in this case, a promise not to complain about Judy's phone calls to her mother. This was, of course, only the first of many interventions into this couple's persistent pattern of blaming one another. Eventually, however, they were able to relate with less anger and more affection.

Challenge the Blamer. A technique borrowed and adapted from a Jay Haley workshop appears to unbalance a rigid blaming system in a constructive way. The therapist chooses one question, which he/she asks one family member throughout an entire session. Any attempt by either party to change the subject is quickly sabotaged by the therapist, who returns the focus to the initial question. When spouses are busy blaming one another the focus on only one question seems to serve at least two purposes: It unbalances the system by emphasizing the behavior of one family member, and it removes the therapist from the position of go-between in negotiating the family's struggle. The following example illustrates one use of this very powerful technique. After 24 years of marriage, Milton and Agnes had a consistent pattern of relating which involved Milton making constant, but obviously long-suffering attempts to please Agnes, who responded by complaining and consistently blaming him for all of her difficulties. Years of therapy with at least a dozen therapists had been unsuccessful in having even a minimal impact on this basic pattern, and had only served to stimulate additional creative variations on their original themes of blame and martyrdom. This particular therapist knew she was clearly stuck in the system when she realized that she was more invested in change than either Milton or Agnes. Agnes blamed Milton for being a Milquetoast, for being passive, for being less than a man. If only he would change, the marriage would have a chance, and the children would be healthy. Milton blamed Agnes because no matter what he did for her, she was dissatisfied. She was unreasonable or mentally ill. Occasionally both of them blamed their past therapists for not helping them sooner. When the couple came into the session in which this "one question" technique was to be used, they began by reporting an incident in which the wife had attacked the husband because their 14-year-old daughter had flushed a sanitary napkin down the toilet, blocking up the plumbing. The question the therapist chose to ask was "Why attack him?" No matter what answer Agnes gave, the question remained "Yes, but why attack him?" Whenever she tried to change the subject, the question was put again: "That's very interesting, but how does that relate to why you attack him?" When other issues were brought up, the therapist said, "Well, yes, but right now, I still want to know why you attack him?" The importance of this question was repeatedly stressed, while no answer was accepted as good enough. As the couple left the session, they were given the assignment of thinking about "Why him?" during the week. When they returned the following week, things were slightly better for the first time in 24 years. Milton had set some limits on his wife's nagging, and Agnes had responded by cooking several of his favorite dishes.

It's unclear why this technique has the power it does. In this case it may have been that the therapist's power reinforced Milton's power to take a stand when the therapist implicitly challenged the legitimacy of Agnes's attacks. It may be that the repeated questioning instilled in Agnes some kind of cognitive delay between the stimulus of something going wrong, and the response of blaming Milton. When she was about to "attack," perhaps she asked herself, "Why him?" making her attack less forceful or making her more receptive to being limited by her husband. In any case, this small change began a series of changes which gradually yet dramatically improved their relationship.

Problem 8. Scapegoating

Scapegoating is another phenomenon which is similar in presentation to both pseudohostility and the blame game. Scapegoating involves the persistent focus upon one member as being the source and location of the family's problems. As a resistance, it can be distinguished from a simple tendency to locate the problem in one member by the persistence with which family members insist on the notion that one member is responsible for all the family's troubles, and on the ferocity of emotion with which they defend this point of view. Again, the true meaning and strength of any resistance can only be gauged by a family's response to the therapist's interventions. Families with a real scapegoat don't move from this position easily, and return to it frequently throughout the course of treatment.

The degree of psychopathology, or at least the behavioral indications that such psychopathology exists within the identified patient, must be taken into consideration when evaluating the meaning of scapegoating. If a severely disturbed person is creating tension by threatening violence, even if the threat seems more manipulation than reality, it is meaningless to decide the family is resisting change by repeatedly scapegoating the identified patient. Something has to be done about the patient's behavior before the family can even begin to consider any changes in the way they treat him.

What is most important to remember about scapegoating is that the victim participates in his/her own martyrdom, either actively provoking the attacks of other family members or passively inviting such attacks by refusing to do anything to help himself/herself. Any efforts made by the therapist to rescue the victim will be resisted as much by the victim as by the rest of the family. In any case, it is wise not to make any immediate and direct attempts to "rescue" the victim. This will only alienate more powerful family members and, since they will not return to therapy, it will help neither the victim nor the family.

SUGGESTIONS

Challenge the Family's Control. There are some cases in which the patient's behavior seems clearly a manifestation of the family system rather than an expression of individual pathology. Remember, for example, Jason's pathetic gestures at overdosing, or Tanya's refusal to learn to inject herself with the insulin she knew she needed in order to survive. In both of these families there was every indication that the identified patient became a scapegoat because the other family members did not know how to control the behavior. Both Jason's parents and Tanya's mother felt overwhelmed by their offspring's behavior. In both these cases, the therapists chose to help the family control the behavior by suggesting specific methods by which they could force the patient to exercise some self-control.

In other families, it seems clear that family members possess the necessary skills to control the behavior they allegedly deplore, but for some reason fail to use these skills. This is particularly true in many families with disturbed adolescents. While these youngsters actually may suffer from disabling feelings of depression, lack of self-esteem, or lack of personal competency, in many cases the family system also allows itself to be manipulated by the symptomatic member. Rather than setting limits on the patient's unreasonable behaviors and encouraging him/her to take responsibility for his/her feelings and behavior, family members respond by allowing themselves to be manipulated and then becoming angry, overprotective or both. In any case, the level of affect usually obscures both other family problems and the strengths and resources the family might have. By leaving the focus on the problem member while intervening to help the family establish some control over the behaviors that are upsetting them, the therapist gains leverage with the family, and lowers affect levels to a point where family energy can be utilized more positively. As a result scapegoating diminishes. This approach is particularly useful with families with very sick members or with those families with severely acting out adolescents or children.

Relabel the Patient's Behavior as Positive or as Serving an Important Function for the Family System. Relabeling the scapegoat's behavior in a positive manner can begin to change the unidimensional view the family has of behavior. For instance, a child's acting out can be relabeled as a sensitive attempt to distract the parents from more painful issues. It is important, in using this technique, to do the relabeling in such a way that the family can accept the message, perhaps simultaneously giving them credit for the positive aspects of the scapegoat's acting out personality. Braulio Montalvo demonstrates a brilliant example of this technique in a Philadelphia Child Guidance Clinic videotape called *The Family with a Little Fire.* In a single-parent family with a young girl who is a fire setter, he not only engages the mother with her daughter around the task of teaching her to light matches safely, but reinforces the child's reading abilities, saying to the mother, "You must have done a lot with her," thus giving the mother credit for the good qualities inherent in the child.

In more strategic terms, the negative behavior of a family member can be relabeled as a sacrifice made for the sake of the family as a whole or for the sake of other family members, if in fact, this is the function it actually seems to play. The Reiss family presented with a 26-year-old son, Ira, who constantly threatened suicide, and kept the family home in consistent turmoil with hostile acting-out behavior. Over a period of several years, he had given up a successful career as an artist, and any attempts to live independently, or to have a social life. His parents did everything for him, including bringing him to therapist after therapist, all of whom were unable to have any impact on his behavior. A family assessment revealed serious underlying marital difficulties and a sadness on the father's part that was nearly disabling. In fact, the only time Mr. Reiss was not depressed was when he was angry about his son. Yet, both parents focused only on Ira's behavior, claiming that if it could be changed, they would be fine. The therapist reframed Ira's behavior in terms of the function it had within the family. Ira, he said, was an extremely sensitive young man who had somehow determined that the family would be harmed or pained were he to leave it. He had, therefore, chosen to make himself a sacrifice for the good of the family, realizing that if he did not, his parents would suffer greatly. The steam went out of Ira's hostility, and his parents' extreme reaction to it. Within a week, Ira had taken a job for the first time in several years.

The Dying Swan. The dying swan is simply another version of a frequently used paradoxical intervention in which the therapist gracefully gives in to the family's resistances by admitting to defeat. Sometimes a therapeutic impasse is resolved by forcing the family to choose between the defeat of the therapist and thus the end of therapy on the one hand, and giving up their resistance on the other. In this intervention, therapists agree that identified patients are what families say they are, "bad," "hopeless," or whatever. Therapists indicate that they, too, cannot think of any solution to the problem and in essence admit that they have been defeated by the magnitude and the stubbornness of the family's problem. Many families respond by instinctively trying to rescue the therapist from this defeat and by trying to prove that their problem is not hopeless. Unaccomplished homework is suddenly completed and difficult tasks become more manageable. A stubborn refusal to budge from the subject of the patient's bad behavior broadens to some self-conceived suggestions of what they might do to improve their own situation. This intervention is best used as a kind of last resort, after all others have failed, and it is not suitable for families with severely disturbed patients unless all other efforts to combat hopelessness have been tried.

Problem 9. Utopian expectations

While unrealistic or utopian expectations do not constitute resistances in and of themselves, they may serve as resistance when they prevent family members from looking at realistic alternatives and accepting the possible rather than the ideal. Most families who have such unrealistic expectations are not even aware that they have any expectations, much less that they are unrealistic. If a family member seems to be stuck in terms of accepting what seem to be reasonable offers of compromise from other family members, it may be helpful to elicit their ideas of the amount of expected conflict in a normal family to see if their ideas are realistic, or to ask what family they would rather be a part of, to see what their fantasies are and what their ideals might be.

SUGGESTIONS

Education. Some families need the help of the therapist in doing a bit of reality testing in order to determine what is reasonable to expect from family life and intimate relationships. This process need not be done in a tedious way through lectures or long explanations. Offhand comments by the therapist can be educative in an important way. To a couple who are disturbed by marital conflict, a therapist might say, "Most couples have quite a bit of conflict, it's a normal part of married life. What is particularly upsetting about this conflict?" Or to parents who are upset at children who have reached an age where they begin to test limits, "It's the job of parents to set limits, it's the job of children to test them. They have to learn just what is acceptable in life and what isn't, to learn whether you mean it. It doesn't mean they don't love you, it means they are normal."

Massive Confrontation. At times, family members so rigidly hold onto their ideals that they look very much like the pseudomutual families described earlier. Alice O'Brien, having bought the Spockian challenge, badly wanted to have raised perfect children. As the children reached adolescence, their normal rebellion and sloppiness seemed to Alice to be a major problem. She brought them to a psychiatric clinic to be "fixed." She had great difficulty accepting the fact that it was impossible to have perfect neatness and perfect harmony in the home. Her husband, Joe, did little to help her to appreciate reality, tending to fade into the woodwork when conflicts arose around their three teenage boys. As part of a more complicated series of interventions, the therapist repeatedly confronted Alice with the normality of her sons, their developmental need for some control of their own boundaries, and the likelihood of much more serious rebellion if they could not establish their separateness in these small ways.

Problem 10. Hopelessness

The opposite problem to that of unreasonable expectations is that of no expectations at all. In such families, family members fail to change at least in part because of their pessimism about the possibility of change. Their genuine hopelessness about life and therapy prevents the possibility of ever moving forward. They believe that even if things changed, they wouldn't be better. They seem to feel as hopeless as the character in the *New Yorker* cartoon who discovered that the light at the end of the tunnel was New Jersey. Pointing out to them their failure to fulfill assigned tasks or to follow through on suggestions yields little, except increased depression, anger, or the admonition that the therapist just doesn't understand.

SUGGESTIONS

Hear Them Out. Sometimes families who remain hopeless about the possibility of change in the midphases of therapy, remain so because of a failure in the joining process early on. If the therapist has not heard all the trials they have been through, the therapies they have tried which have failed, family members are likely to feel that the therapist does not truly grasp the severity of their problem. Therefore, when the therapist gives reassurance, it seems false and unbelievable. When the therapist assigns tasks, they seem unattainable. In such cases, therefore, it helps to return to a detailed review of what they have been through, including a careful examination of all past attempts at change. This review will also help the therapist to devise a strategy that will be somewhat different from those used in the past.

Give Them Hope. If the therapist has heard the details of a family's problems, and has established himself/herself as an expert in the family's eyes, the therapist may be able to give hope by building on his/her own expertise and experience. The therapist can say, "This is a very serious problem, and I can see why you are so discouraged, but you have been working hard. I have treated many families with this problem, and although it has taken a lot of work on your part, I can promise you that things will be better soon." If the hopelessness is encountered in the latter stages of therapy, the therapist may want to emphasize that things often look worse just before they really begin to improve, which happens to be true.

The Swan Dies Again. Hopeless families are very much like families who maintain a rigid focus on the identified patient. In fact, one indication of hopelessness is an inability to see the problem from any other perspective or to expand the focus. If a situation is not truly impossible, but rather the hopelessness seems to be serving some function in the system, such as preventing people from using their resources to deal with their problems, it may be helpful to go along with the hopelessness. The therapist in so many words says, "You have a lot to be depressed about." For example, the Steins were a middle-class family who had a son, a chronic gambler, who had already lost one job because he had stolen from the store which employed him. He also stole from his own family, writing bad checks on his parents' accounts. Despite the therapist's efforts to get his parents to set some limits on these behaviors, they were caught in a web of hopelessness. They absolutely couldn't follow through on the therapist's "radical" suggestion that they require David to take responsibility for his behavior. The therapist finally accepted their notion that the situation was hopeless, that as good parents they could not bring charges against their son, or for that matter, refuse to pay off on the bad checks he wrote so that the stores which honored the checks would take legal action. The therapist resorted to nodding agreement with their "Let me tell you how bad it is" statements and apologized for not being able to help them, saying how sad it was that David would have to get into even more serious trouble before he would stop himself. The therapist was also vague about scheduling another appointment telling the Steins to get in touch with her "later." Mrs. Stein called a few weeks later to say that after finding out that David had

not attended a meeting of Gamblers Anonymous which he had promised
to attend, she had gone along with her husband's suggestion that they
throw him out. David's father confiscated his key and gave him only a
small satchel of clothes. David, of course, immediately found refuge with
his grandparents, but his parents were able to insist he would not be allowed to come home unless he found a job, attended GA, and paid off all
the money they had spent covering his bad checks. It would be nice to be
able to report that David stopped gambling. He did not, but his parents re-
gained some sense of control and self-esteem, and he did stop stealing
from them.

Problem 11. Family privacy, family secrets, and withholding information

Family secrets constitute resistance in family therapy when they fall
into one of four categories: when family members have secrets from each
other which interfere with the free and open use of the family therapy sessions; when they have secrets from each other which they attempt to share
with the therapist without sharing them with each other; when they have
secrets which they share with each other but not with the therapist; or
when they are afraid that the therapist will share their secrets with the
world.

Many families are very sensitive about the issue of family privacy,
feeling that they should not "wash their dirty laundry in public." Public
often includes the therapist as well. The family boundary is rigidly maintained, and crossing it is viewed by family members as a betrayal of the
family's integrity. Some families have such a high value on family privacy
that they cannot use therapy at all, while others are simply ambivalent. In
either case, therapy is difficult.

Secrets may involve facts about the family's history such as past de-
pressions, mental illnesses, or suicide attempts. On the other hand, secrets
may involve more current events such as one family member having an extramarital affair or a young person taking drugs without parental knowledge. Sometimes withholding information involves a collusion between
the mother and child to keep the father out of the family life, and at times,
to keep the therapist out as well. The mother does not tell the father or
therapist about the child's misbehavior because she feels the response will
be negative. Other family members encourage withholding of past psychiatric history from the therapist or behaviors they feel would be socially unacceptable such as child or wife abuse. A therapist should usually suspect
that information is being withheld when nothing changes regardless of the
interventions used. Appropriate intervention on the issue of secrets depends on the function of the secret in the family and how the family or its
member is using it with the therapist.

For example, if the secret is a terminated extramarital affair, it may or may not be important to ask the family member to share this information with the spouse. Family therapy need not require that all family members relinquish their rights to privacy in all areas of their life simply because they have elected family treatment. True confessions about affairs may cause more difficulty than they resolve, stimulating a focus on the affair as a red herring and directing attention from the marriage. If, on the other hand, an extramarital affair is in process, it is usually important that it be terminated or revealed because it will drain the energy and commitment of a family member's work in therapy, and put the therapist in the position of colluding with one spouse against the other. In this way it may function as an obstacle to the usefulness of the sessions and the resolution of marital problems.

These issues become further complicated when family members attempt to engage the therapist in maintaining secrets from other family members through the use of "door knobbers," that is, hanging behind departing family members to tell the therapist something about the family, or calling between family sessions asking that the phone call or its content not be shared with other family members. In such instances, a therapist can be caught in collusions which tie his/her hands and prevent effective intervention, or stimulate a lack of trust on the part of other family members.

SUGGESTIONS

Support the Privacy Value. One method of dealing with the issue of excessively guarded family privacy which keeps the therapist out, is to agree with the family's value of family privacy, while stressing the need for openness in therapy in order to insure that family privacy is maintained. For example, as one of our colleagues has suggested, the therapist may say, "I agree with you that this should not be stated in public and therefore, we had better deal with it right now before the school, the police, and other institutions become involved in this process."

Ask Them to Imagine Having Told the Secret. When secrets are being kept between family members, a good method of easing into dealing with the real issues (lack of trust, fear of rejection, etc.) is to ask family members to imagine having told a secret and then to discuss the reaction they would expect to receive from various family members. The therapist can emphasize that the secret itself is less important than their fear of the responses they would receive from other family members in the process.

Avoid Collusions and Triangulation. When family members attempt to engage the therapist in a contract to keep secrets from other family members, bells should toll, and at least one red flag should wave vigorously. Therapists should avoid such bargains at all costs. This is not to say that they should repeat everything they hear from every family member. It is to say that therapists should maintain control over what they will tell whom. Otherwise, they are vulnerable to triangulation, blackmail, and hopeless muddles. Therapists must communicate to family members who wish private conferences, even very brief ones, that if they feel any information is important to the family that they will ask that the member share that information in the next session.

Three final interventions for all seasons

"Try It for Just One Week." A "when everything else has failed" gambit involves the therapist pointing out that change is not irreversible, that the family can always go back to their old way of doing things, but that they should agree to do things the therapist's way for a specified period of time. Of course, the danger is that the family may well sabotage any interventions made in this way if they feel they have a vested interest in defeating the therapist. If they do not, they may be pleasantly surprised by the changes produced by suggestions made by the therapist. Some people resist the therapist's interventions because they really think something won't work or that the therapist just doesn't understand the situation. Sometimes they are right. Knowing they can go back to their old ways and that a trial doesn't mean a commitment gives them some freedom to experiment.

The Cohen family was unable to cope with their 25-year-old daughter's psychotic behavior. Despite the fact that Phyllis was unreasonable, belligerent, and imposed bizarre rituals on the rest of the family, they felt unable to set any limits on her behavior because she was "sick." The therapist's attempts to explain her need for structure and control were to no avail, as the family continued to allow her to determine the rules of the household. Her parents could not believe it was possible that she could control her behavior or that she would not be damaged and rejected by their regaining control of the family. Finally, the therapist resorted to choosing one objectionable behavior and asking the parents to establish a rule about that behavior for just one week. If, at the end of that week, it seemed too difficult for them, or their daughter was unable to adjust to the new rule, the therapist agreed to stop pressuring the family about the issue. The parents chose to set a rule about food. For years, every two to three days, Phyllis had arbitrarily chosen to throw away most of the food in the house, saying it was contaminated. With much trepidation, for the first time the parents told Phyllis that this behavior was unacceptable. She did not have to eat any food she felt was contaminated, but she could not decide this issue for the entire family. A week later, Phyllis not only had accepted the rule, but seemed pleased that her parents had set it. The parents were shocked that she responded so positively, and had new hope for change, and increased confidence that they might have the power to improve their lives.

Use Networks (in the Sessions or by Long Distance). When a family is in crisis or is feeling at the end of their rope, exhausted and without resources, it is often useful to activate their extended family or their immediate social network. This can be done by inviting this entire group to a meeting, or by involving them with one another outside the sessions. Many therapists shy away from network therapy because of the intimidating number of people involved. However, a family's network need not all be in the room at the same time to be helpful. For example, Kitty, a young mother of two, became acutely paranoid and psychotic, and refused to talk with her therapist whom she now believed to be part of a plot against her. She had religious delusions in which she believed that she had to purify her home by throwing all her furniture and her clothing, and that of her children, out of the window of her apartment into the snow below. A network consisting of her mother and sisters, several neighbors, her stepfather, and her real father was convened to convince her to accept treatment. These network members came to the hospital for sessions on how to be helpful, or made themselves available by phone. Using combinations of relatives, the therapist was able to arrange for the care of Kitty's children to be transferred to her mother, and to remove a handgun she had in her apartment. While it was impossible to convince her to come to the hospital as she feared involuntary admission, it was possible to stabilize the situation and prevent her from harming herself or the children.

Shake Things Up. When nothing rational has worked and the therapist is desperate, it's sometimes good to make a change, any change, particularly when the therapist suspects that he/she may have become an integral part of the forces maintaining the status quo in a given family. Even though both therapist and family may be enjoying the sessions, and sometimes the process of therapy is interesting and/or fun, therapy is not legitimate unless it is moving toward the changes required by the family. If a good family therapy consultant is available, so much the better, but if not, the therapist may try a change in the frequency of sessions, or introduce any new strategy of intervention which could shake things loose from the therapeutic impasse, and get therapy moving again. The therapist may wish to discuss the fact that things are becoming too comfortable for everyone, and thus make the family a part of the decision to try something new. On the other hand, the therapist may wish to employ a new technique without giving a reason to the family, allowing the new technique to serve as a diagnostic tool, revealing to therapists how they have become caught in the family system. In either case, the point is to make any change that will challenge the status quo, the assumptions on which everyone has come to operate, and the rules of therapy that have failed to maintain pressure for change.

Summary

Resistance in ongoing therapy is defined as all behaviors, feelings, patterns, or styles that operate to prevent change. Resistances may appear in many forms: They may be overt or covert, may be conscious or unconscious, and may appear to reside in one family member, or appear to be distributed throughout the family system. In fact, resistance usually moves from overt to covert states, and moves from one part of the system to another. Regardless of the form it takes, what is important about any behavior defined as resistance is its function in preventing change. Sequences are the key to understanding the function, meaning, and strength of any resistance and the best way to deal with it.

Every therapist must learn to look to the patterns and sequences of behaviors surrounding any one behavior in order to judge whether it is best to directly challenge the behavior, ignore it, or employ some other means of handling it. The therapist's theoretical orientation is the greatest determinant of what behaviors will be seen as resistance. This is because resistance does not reside in a family per se, but is a product of the interaction between the therapist and the family. (Action-oriented therapists and insight-oriented therapists will consider different behaviors resistant.) This chapter has described a number of common resistances in ongoing treatment, along with a variety of suggested interventions to be used in coping with them.

6. Resistances produced by helping systems

We have met the enemy and they are us.—POGO

Carlos Sluzki tells a story about a young man who was attacked by a jaguar while walking in a jungle in Latin America. He pulled out his gun and shot the jaguar at the last minute, saving his own life. He told his adventure to a friend who became very excited. "My God," the friend said, "What would you have done if you didn't have a gun with you?" The young man thought a moment and then said, "Well, I guess I would have pulled out my machete and stabbed him." "Yes, yes," the friend said, "but what if you didn't have your machete, what would you have done then?" The young man thought again, then said, "I guess I would have grabbed a big stick and hit him with it." "Well good, but what if you couldn't have found a big stick fast enough, what would you have done then?" "Well," said the young man, "I guess I would have tried to climb a tree." "Yes, but," said the friend, "what if you couldn't or there was no tree big enough, what then?" The young man stopped short, "Wait just a minute here," he said to his friend, "are you a friend of mine or a friend of the jaguar's?"

This story illustrates the feeling of many family therapists as they try to do therapy within the context of a helping system of one sort or another. The system that is supposed to support them sometimes seems to be more the friend of the jaguar, or in this case, the friend of resistance. As if it were not enough for therapists to have to deal with the varied forms of resistance brought by the families they treat, therapists are also confronted with some subtle and not so subtle resistances to family therapy in themselves, in the institutions in which they work, and in the systems which have the power to decide what type of psychotherapy and/or psychotherapist will receive financial support.

In Chapter 1, the point was made that resistance could be viewed as a property of the therapeutic system, that is, as residing in the family or its members, the therapist, and/or the systems within which therapists practice. Viewed in this way, resistance can be seen to operate in an interactive, cumulative, and even synergistic way as the resistance of the family contributes to the resistance of the therapist and so on.

207

A look at how resistance interacts within various components of the therapeutic system can be seen in the following case example.

Eighteen-year-old Sylvia was hospitalized after making a suicidal gesture by taking her mother's antidepressant medication. The routine intake interview revealed that Sylvia's mother, Glenna, had been depressed since her divorce from Sylvia's father and the institutionalization of her drug-abusing son. During this same time period Sylvia had graduated from high school, and had gone to college at one of the rural campuses of the state university, where she had flourished, dating for the first time. As the first semester progressed, Sylvia's mother, perhaps because she became somewhat less depressed and self-involved, initiated a series of subtle messages to her daughter indicating that she wished she would come home. Sylvia became increasingly withdrawn and depressed, finally returning home immediately after the spring term. She took her mother's medication almost at once. The inpatient unit to which Sylvia was admitted focused on both the potential biochemical aspects of her depression and the potential impact of family issues. The inpatient family therapist attempted to focus on the process of Sylvia's emancipation from home, and how this process had been complicated for both Sylvia and Glenna by other family events. Both mother and daughter were resistant to discussing these issues. Nevertheless, they formed an attachment to the family therapist whom they viewed as having been helpful during a family crisis, and only reluctantly accepted the necessity of a change of therapists for outpatient family therapy when Sylvia was discharged. Although a transitional interview, which included both therapists, was arranged, the inpatient therapist did not tell the outpatient therapist that Glenna and Sylvia had been resistant to discussing problematic issues. When Glenna and Sylvia claimed that they had found their sessions with her useful, she let it go at that. She was worried that her difficulties in handling the family might be viewed as a lack of skill on her part. The outpatient therapist noted some family resistance in the session, but attributed it to a natural reluctance to change therapists and set up an appointment to meet with the family the following week.

Glenna called the day of the appointment, announcing that she had received a huge bill from the hospital. She didn't know if her insurance would cover the bill, and her call to the hospital's billing department left her with the impression that sorting out the problem was up to her. In the meantime she stated, she couldn't afford to increase her financial liability with more therapy. She claimed that therapy was unnecessary anyway, since Sylvia was doing fine. The outpatient therapist knew she was dealing with a normal resistance to changing therapists that was probably surmountable. She also knew she could run interference with the billing department for Glenna, or make a case for the importance of after care, but she did not. She was already overextended with too many patients and she was irritated at the need to deal with a billing department that seemed to continuously make errors in billing family therapy cases. She told Glenna she was glad things were going so well and that she should feel free to call if she ever changed her mind about therapy.

In this example, Glenna's and Sylvia's natural resistance to making the changes necessary for Sylvia to successfully emancipate was exacerbated by three distinct systems-based factors which made it easy for them to avoid further family therapy. Each of these systems issues operates as a resistance to involving and treating families successfully. The first systems factor was the lack of coordination, cooperation, and trust between inpatient and outpatient systems as represented by two family therapists. Each system viewed the other with suspicion; neither gave the other much support or credit. The second systems factor was contributed by the billing department. While bills are inevitable, this particular bill included neither an explanation of the charges, nor an explanation of how much Glenna was responsible for and how much the insurance would pay. Further, the billing department did have a history of making frequent errors in billing for family therapy and of becoming irritable and defensive when families and therapists challenged their accuracy. While this bill was not in error, the reputation of the billing department caused most clinicians in the system to avoid contact with them if at all possible. The third systems factor was the outpatient therapist's failure to pursue Glenna's reasons for withdrawing, preferring to accept the loss of the case, rather than putting the energy into straightening out the billing issue, and handling any other expressions of resistance by Glenna and Sylvia. In her heart, she knew she could have done more to involve this family and that their resistance was surmountable, but it was relatively easy to label the family as uncooperative and dismiss them. Her message to Glenna was clear, don't call back until you're really ready to work!

Although this was indeed a resistant family, this example clearly demonstrates how the behaviors and feelings of various parts of helping systems can operate as resistances to conducting successful treatment. In this case, these factors interacted to result in the failure of a family to enter treatment. If any one of these behaviors had not occurred, if the inpatient worker had prepared the outpatient therapist for the family's resistance, if the bill had been more understandable, had come at another time, or if the billing department had had a better reputation, or if the outpatient therapist had been less fatigued, then perhaps it would have been possible to encourage the family to stay in treatment long enough to overcome their own resistances. While the people in this case failed to engage in outpatient family therapy, an awareness of the potential problems stimulated by systems resistances may help to avoid or surmount them in similar cases.

This chapter will discuss resistances residing in the clinician, in the system in which he/she works, and, briefly, in those systems which govern the ways in which health care and social services are delivered. While the discussion is not meant to be comprehensive, since every therapist, agency, and institution has its own idiosyncratic quirks, an attempt will be made to demonstrate some of the ways the behaviors and policies of professionals unwittingly function as resistances to family therapy in helping systems. Although these "resistances" are arbitrarily divided for the sake of clarity, it must be understood that they occur simultaneously and interact with each other in ways which decrease the likelihood that successful therapy will be conducted.

Resistances of therapists

Resistances within therapists consist of those thoughts, feelings, and behaviors which contribute to a failure to engage with or treat families successfully. These thoughts, feelings, and behaviors occur with all family therapists, but may be exacerbated by being a beginner, being coerced to do family therapy, being a victim of therapist fatigue, or all of the above.

Beginners in family therapy are either clinicians with experience in other models of psychotherapy or novices to the field. They are learning family therapy voluntarily and enthusiastically, or with some degree of skepticism and/or coercion. The system in which they practice may support this learning process or discourage it. All of these variables will influence the amount of enthusiasm or ambivalence therapists bring with them to their initial experiences with families. Even under optimum conditions, some degree of therapist resistance is to be expected simply because it is uncomfortable to learn a new modality of treatment. Even those students who beg for placements in agencies where they can learn family therapy find themselves expressing resistance once they are actually on the front line. A colleague of ours confessed that despite her initial motivation to learn family therapy, she was so nervous when she received her first referral that she called the family three times, each time hanging up after the first ring. She solemnly reported to her supervisor that she had tried several times to reach them and they didn't answer their phone.

The resistance of beginning family therapists wears many faces, few as overt as that of our colleague who hung up the phone after one ring. It is usually not deliberate opposition to family therapy. Rather, it is most likely to be caused by competence anxiety, which can be exacerbated by inadequate supervision; ambivalence about the efficacy of family therapy, which can be exacerbated by lack of experience; or therapist fatigue, which can be exacerbated by lack of skill.

Competence anxiety

Most therapists learning a new modality are concerned about feeling and looking incompetent. Competence anxiety is nearly universal and has nothing to do with a lack of commitment to learning and practicing a family approach. Nobody likes to appear incompetent, even if it is a necessary stage of learning. Total novices to the practice of psychotherapy are further disadvantaged by the lack of any clinical experience with the role of therapist. Their competence anxiety is complicated by the overwhelming sense of responsibility most new therapists feel for their patients.

The situation is in some ways better and some ways worse for therapists experienced in other therapeutic modalities. While they are likely to know at least something about human behavior, the role of the therapist, and the ground rules of therapy, they must relinquish a role in which they have established competence to place themselves in the position of being learners. The insecurities inherent in giving up a comfortable role for an unknown and untested one, compounded by the need to accept supervision, can result in resentment and therapeutic failures.

While most therapists are aware of their concerns about their own competence, most are not aware of how these concerns lead them to participate in creating or exacerbating the resistance of families. Most therapists tend to see resistance as residing totally within families. They are initially quite mystified when they are told that they can transmit their own insecurities and anxieties to the family directly during a phone call. They are unaware that a family's failure to show up for an initial appointment may be related to their own timid tone of voice when they arranged the session, or their communication of a lack of confidence in a variety of messages they have sent. They waffle when family members ask about their training, or when family members question whether family therapy is really the most effective method of therapeutic interventions for a particular problem. They may even find themselves covertly, or even overtly, agreeing with family members that the problem so clearly resides in only one family member that the idea of family sessions is ludicrous.

Therapists fears of appearing and feeling incompetent are often complicated by common family therapy training procedures such as the use of videotape and/or live supervision. Beginning family therapists must expose their practice to the eyes of others at a time when they are struggling to make sense of a whole different perspective on why people behave as they do and how to change the ways in which they behave. Exposing their work at such times is difficult for young and inexperienced therapists. It is even more difficult for therapists who are experienced in other modalities and who thus must simultaneously relinquish tried and true practices.

The competence anxiety of beginning family therapists also can be complicated by logistical issues which further the cause of therapist resistance. The difficulty in convening family meetings, the need for larger spaces, flexible hours, and experienced supervision may seem insurmountable problems to ambivalent beginners. One of our students faced two of these problems in her first position as a therapist. Her office was too small for her to use to see families, and her supervisor was unfamiliar with family therapy. Undaunted, she asked if she could pursue a family approach. She was given permission to try, but in order to do so she had to borrow a bigger office. Since senior personnel tend to have the biggest offices, she found herself borrowing her supervisor's office, thus inconveniencing a supervisor who didn't even practice the form of therapy she was attempting to learn. A less secure beginner might have given up seeing families, considering the logistical difficulties and the lack of experienced supervision.

Although this student persevered without supervision, therapist resistance usually is also related both to the availability of supervision and the behaviors of the supervisor. Therapists untrained in family therapy quite sensibly balk, or at least have some trepidation, about seeing families without knowledgeable and skillful guidance. While a supervisor with knowledge about families and skill in family therapy is certainly desirable for novices, the support of a supervisor would seem to be a bare minimum. Supervisors who give half-hearted support for the modality tend to produce students who learn only how to lose families in the early stages of therapy. Beginners without support are almost certainly destined to fail. In summary, one type of therapist resistance to family therapy is a manifestation of clinician anxiety, inept supervision, or a combination of both. The situation described above of a student without experienced supervision was one ripe to encourage family resistance and to set in motion a spiraling process in which family therapy is likely to fail or be abandoned as a legitimate modality.

Therapist ambivalence about the efficacy of family therapy

When they begin to see families, both beginners and therapists experienced in other treatment modalities are skeptical about the practice of family therapy. Beginners tend to focus on the manipulative qualities of some models of family intervention, their "ethical" need to tell family members everything they observe and think, and their inability to really believe in the connection between one individual's symptomatology and the way the rest of the family behaves. While these variables are of concern to therapists completely new to the practice of psychotherapy, the problem is much more complicated for therapists experienced in other treatment modalities but new to family work. Their skepticism about family therapy is exacerbated by being confronted with a radically changed view of what behaviors are required in order for them to be effective as therapists. For instance, the psychodynamic model of individual therapy is conceptually complicated, sophisticated, and takes a long time to learn. This in itself would be sufficient incentive for a psychodynamically oriented therapist to hold to that modality above all others. But there are also things about the way that therapy is conducted that can make the transition to family therapy difficult. The overt behavior required of the individual therapist is relatively uncomplicated. The work of understanding is behind the scenes. Patience, awareness, and the use of transference are difficult skills to learn, but therapists are usually not observed when they practice these skills and they rarely look foolish if they can't think on their feet. Even if they make errors, only they and perhaps their patients are aware of it. While they may be supervised, certainly their supervisors don't watch or intervene in sessions. The method of treatment and supervision has the built-in protections of pace, privacy, and therapist inactivity.

Family therapy is different in just about every way. Current theories are not complicated once one has grasped a few basic systems notions such as the concepts of boundaries, hierarchies, and circular causality. However, the overt behavior required of a competent family therapist in a family session is complex, extremely difficult to learn, and usually blatantly exposed. Therapists must be much more active and controlling than therapists are in sessions with individuals, and must take more responsibility for change. While individual therapists must be aware of processes of therapist–patient interaction, the increased number of people in family sessions requires that family therapists must recognize and assimilate more data than the individual therapist, and must do so more rapidly.

Essentially, in family therapy therapists must learn to function as human computers, observing a multifaceted system of complex behavior patterns, while making, testing, and accepting or rejecting ever evolving hypotheses about families. They are constantly modifying their view of a family and its members, all the while monitoring their responses to interventions. Furthermore, family therapists must accomplish this feat in front of everyone in the family, and often also in front of videocameras or a one-way mirror. It is not surprising that therapists new to the field would have doubts about the efficacy of such procedures and be reluctant to expose themselves and families to them. Worries about confidentiality, manipulation, and the impact of short-term contracts all contribute to therapists' tendencies to display behaviors that function as resistances to family therapy. These resistances in therapists new to family work are not aided by the drama and religious fervor in the family therapy field. Demonstration interviews, workshops, and writings by family experts seem to many newcomers to suggest interventions they could not possibly assimilate, to oversimplify the complex nature of change and therapy, and thus increase skepticism about the efficacy of the approach.

Therapist fatigue

A special form of therapist resistance may be created or exacerbated in both beginning and experienced therapists by "therapist fatigue." Therapists who are suffering from therapist fatigue tend to feel a sense of relief when families cancel, to experience decreased energy for family sessions, to lack interest in the outcome of therapy, and to have persistent ruminations over whether they have chosen the right profession. Therapists suffering from this syndrome postpone or fail altogether to return phone calls from families, are slow to reschedule cancelled sessions, tend to see the same dynamics in every case and repeatedly state that the prognosis is "guarded." In more advanced cases of this syndrome, therapists may also find themselves missing work frequently with minor health complaints.

Therapist fatigue usually is caused by long-term responsibility for too many difficult cases, too little support from fellow clinicians or administration, and/or too little variety in one's work and life. This syndrome, known by many different names is most popularly called "burn out." The authors prefer the term "fatigue" because it implies a temporary condition which can be alleviated, while "burn out" implies that therapists are permanently and completely "used up." If fatigue is not relieved, however, it may become chronic and result in irreversible "burn out," a condition in which therapists develop a generalized resistance to doing family treatment. Unless they have an unusual amount of support, beginning family therapists are more vulnerable to therapist fatigue than veterans because they lack the cushion of a history of positive reinforcement from succesful cases.

Common expressions of therapist resistance

Therapists tend to express their resistance to family therapy by failing to attend to the details necessary to get family therapy or family therapy supervision off the ground or keep it going; by accepting natural surmountable family resistances as legitimate reasons to put off or discontinue therapy; or by actually overtly or covertly encouraging families to discontinue treatment.

The first set of these therapist resistances relates to mundane details. Arranging for appropriate office space, agreeing to work in the evening, or arranging to videotape are all key areas in which a therapist's resistance to doing or learning family therapy can be expressed. Resistant therapists tend to refuse to see families that can't get in before five in the afternoon. They also rarely manage to videotape their family sessions. Most frequently they report that their families simply refuse to be videotaped, but variations on this theme include such excuses as camera dysfunction, broken playback machines, the inability to find a usable tape, or the inability to get families to come in when the taping room is available.

The second set of therapist behaviors that operate as resistances relate to the therapist's too easy acceptance of family resistances. The therapist's response to Glenna and Sylvia was of this type. When they were resistant to therapy, the therapist gave in to this resistance with no attempt to use her skills to establish a therapeutic alliance and involve them in therapy. Since the vast majority of families coming to treatment are ambivalent about committing themselves to this process, therapists who side with the negative side of the ambivalence will lose most families before the first session.

The third set of therapist behaviors that operate as resistances are those which involve overt or covert encouragement for families to discontinue treatment even when resistance is not particularly active in families at the time. Therapists who are resistant in this way tend to "dump" cases using a variety of excuses; the family is too difficult to treat, there is no hope for the marriage, the family is uncommitted. They may directly tell the family that treatment is not indicated, or they may use a more subtle approach. For example, one of the authors was referred a couple in which the husband was labeled as having a "paranoid jealousy syndrome." It had been her experience that such cases are extremely difficult to treat in couples therapy. Not only is violence an ever present threat, but if therapists are not firmly and consistently directive and on top of things, family sessions quickly become unstructured and further stimulate jealous ruminations causing the individual and the marriage to get worse. Nevertheless, in this case, after several sessions, there had been surprisingly little overt resistance on the part of the couple. They had become immediately dependent on the therapist and consistently used her in their many crises. In the fourth session, the husband mentioned that it had been helpful when his old individual therapist had told him he was not allowed to hit his wife. While this was probably a message to the therapist requesting even more limits and structure, the therapist responded with a few questions about his individual therapy and ended up suggesting that maybe he shouldn't have given it up. The husband brought her up short, interrupting by saying, "Wait just a minute here, are you trying to get rid of me?" He was absolutely right. She was resisting treating this couple because it was difficult and taxed her time and energies. Fortunately, this patient was paranoid enough to call her on her evasion and she was able to get control of her own resistance in time to continue with the case.

When therapists are truly skeptical about family therapy they may adopt what can be called the St. George approach, setting up a series of ever more difficult dragons to be slain. Their own resistance to the modality causes them to select cases which are so intractable that the founding fathers and mothers of family therapy together couldn't produce change.

When family therapy fails to have an impact, they say to themselves, "I knew family therapy wouldn't work," and return to their old methods of practice, claiming, and believing, that they have given the modality a fair chance.

In summary, whether therapist resistance is the result of competence anxiety, ambivalence about the efficacy and morality of the practice of family therapy, or the result of therapist fatigue, resistance is usually projected onto the family. Therapist must learn to recognize that they may be playing an important role in initiating, perpetuating, or exacerbating family resistance.

Resistances of agencies and institutions

Sometimes the primary location of resistance is neither in the family nor the therapist, but in the larger system in which the therapist practices. These larger systems resistances can be caused by lack of exposure to family therapy, institutional *diablos conocidos,* or the system's response to the unwitting provocations of family therapists.

Resistances in agencies and institutions can usefully be divided into those which reside principally in the clinical staff and those which reside in the administration, although in smaller agencies these functions are often carried out by the same persons. The reason for this division is that resistances residing in clinical staff tend to be related to unfamiliarity with family therapy and its underlying assumptions, while resistances residing in administration tend to be associated with the unusual demands family therapists make on the systems in which they operate. Both reflect a lack of commitment to the practice of family therapy.

Lack of exposure by senior clinicians

Professionals are loyal to those methods in which they are trained, comfortable, and with which they have experienced success. Many senior supervisors and administrators of agencies or clinics received their training before family therapy was included as an integral part of training programs. They are not necessarily hostile toward family therapy, but they do lack an understanding of its theories, methods, goals, and potential benefits. Much of what looks like resistance to family therapy by helping systems, therefore, is due to unfamiliarity with or lack of acceptance of the idea of producing change in a symptomatic person by manipulating the context of the symptom. In fact, many traditionally oriented senior clinicians would flinch at the thought of any kind of "manipulation" as a therapeutic approach.

Institutional resistance due to lack of familiarity with family therapy usually manifests itself passively as an absence of policies which consider family needs and family issues, a reluctance to discuss the relevance of family therapy to the overall clinical care program, and/or a skepticism as to the efficacy of this modality, particularly when it comes to difficult cases. Even clinicians who are usually supportive of family therapy have been heard to say, "This case is really tough. It needs individual therapy," as if family therapy were appropriate only when the symptoms aren't too serious. This sort of remark may reflect hostility toward a family point of view, but more often it represents the natural inclination of clinicians to resort to methods in which they have been trained, in which they have experienced success, and which they understand.

Sometimes senior clinicians avoid discussions of family issues because they simply don't want to reveal how unfamiliar they are with family theory. One of the authors learned that lesson shortly after joining the staff of the department of psychiatry of a large teaching hospital. She worked for weeks on her first Grand Rounds presentation, painfully editing hours of videotape into a 20-minute presentation of the effects of chronic illness on an otherwise functional family, attempting to demonstrate how certain interventions could be made to help family members cope more effectively. Following the presentation the floor was opened for the usual discussion by faculty members and psychiatric residents. First there was an uncomfortable silence, then a few questions about the patient's diagnosis (end-stage renal disease), followed by speculation about how long the patient could survive on dialysis. Despite her repeated attempts to refocus the discussion, no one commented on family issues, and no one mentioned her strategies of intervention even though these had been demonstrated by a large chart and sections of videotape. After the presentation was over, she asked a colleague what had gone wrong. "Nothing," she was told, "most people around here don't know a lot about family therapy, so they talk about what they know. We're making progress, though. At least they don't say, 'Family what?' anymore."

Lack of familiarity with family therapy is sometimes complicated by the fact that some senior clinicians may assume they know what family therapy is all about when they do not. Negative reactions are not uncommon when they find that their assumptions are wrong. For example, a physician referred his brother to the family therapy clinic for treatment of a marital problem. He withdrew his support and caused a premature end to treatment when he learned that his brother and sister-in-law were talking to each other in sessions rather than his sister-in-law talking to the therapist about her mother, which was what he had in mind. This referring physician rightly believed that his brother's wife had unresolved issues with her mother. He wrongly believed that this was the only cause of the couple's marital problems, and that the family therapist would simply tell the wife to deal with her mother. He certainly did not understand that their particular family therapist would assume current problems are maintained by current contexts and thus conduct therapy which focused on the present, even if the etiology of some of their marital problems did relate to the wife's relationship with her mother. Exposure to the concept of circular causality was not a part of his training.

Institutional *diablos conocidos*

Standard agency procedures are to helping systems what *diablos conocidos* are to family systems. They are habitual procedures that have worked in the past. They are proven to be effective and efficient, and consistent with the belief systems of both the power structure of the agency and the clinicians who do the work. Such a system will resist changing its practices to incorporate a treatment modality or a therapist that they do not understand or with which they are not familiar. Usually they will attempt to incorporate the model without making changes in any basic policies. Family therapy, however, is revolutionary. A family approach, consistently applied, requires changes all down the line.

Institutions in our culture focus on the individual as a unit about which they collect information and keep records for many very practical reasons. In our transient, ever changing culture, families divide and multiply in unpredictable ways. It's much easier to keep track of people one at a time. However, this institutional focus on the individual greatly influences the kind of information that is sought and recorded, and thus the kind of treatment it is possible to do. In health care systems, the kind of information collected about the patient and his/her problem influences the choice of interventions it will make to try to help. For instance, unless patients present their complaints in terms of family issues, they are usually not asked to discuss their problems in relationship to their family situation. In this way, systems may be insensitive to family issues or resistant to family interventions because their general individually based policies fail to collect the information necessary to understand a given case from a family perspective. For example, Anna, a woman suffering from depression, presented herself at the emergency room of a psychiatric hospital. She talked of things being hopeless, of life having no meaning, of her sense of worthlessness. In such a situation, unless the clinician doing the evaluation asked more than a routine question about family issues, he/she would not hear about them because this depressed woman believed she was to blame for everything negative that had ever happened to her. Nevertheless, Anna's depression had begun after she discovered her husband's extramarital affair which occurred simultaneously with the loss of her ongoing support systems through a geographically long-distance move.

Most clinicians operating strictly on a medical model would look first to symptom relief in such cases. Anna received a workup to reassure the clinician that the depression was not the result of some undiagnosed medical condition and, since she had changes in her vegetative functions (sleep, appetite, sexual interest), she was given a trial on antidepressant medication. Only when her husband encouraged her noncompliance with a medication regime did the clinician look beyond the individual patient to family issues. By this time, Anna, her family, and the health care delivery system had focused so intently on Anna as the only problem, that it was difficult for anyone to persuade her family that their behaviors also had an important effect.

Systems resistances caused by therapist attitudes

Some systems may become resistant to family therapy due to the attitude of family therapists. Therapists who are committed to the family model as the most efficient and efficacious model of treatment, to the point of becoming "true believers," can antagonize their colleagues by claiming to possess the Truth and the Light. Other staff, who feel they have managed to help a few people over the years, are put off by this attitude of smug superiority. While the true believer approach is unwise in most instances, it is particularly unwise for family therapists just beginning to operate in traditional settings established and maintained on a medical model. The relative youth of the family therapy movement makes it likely that the clinicians in any system who are most likely to want to practice family therapy are relatively new to the system and therefore low in the power structure. Thus, a family therapist who takes on a whole system in a head-on power struggle is not only likely to lose, but to emerge from such a battle at best with a premature case of therapist fatigue, or at worst without a job.

Problems between the "true believer" in family therapy and the rest of the clinical staff usually concern the issue of turf. With all of its problems, the old multidisciplinary team had the advantage of clear-cut roles and divisions of responsibility. Traditionally, the physician was regarded as having jurisdiction over all matters concerning the patient, psychologists were responsible for assessing patients through the use of projective tests, while another member of the team, usually a nurse or social worker, dealt with the family. The introduction of family therapy muddied the waters by making the family a more integral part of treatment. When the family became the patient, who took the responsibility for the family therapy became more a matter of interest and training than of professional discipline. It can as easily be a physician, psychologist, social worker, or nurse. Clear-cut boundaries between roles and responsibilities have become blurred, and turf issues have had to be renegotiated.

How well the negotiations go between staff of various orientations depends on how flexible everyone is willing to be. Family therapists are not the only true believers. Staff who are devoted to the psychodynamic model may insist that the patient be viewed and treated as an individual, taking a rigid position against family therapy. Staff who are devoted to a biological model may view family therapy as an irrelevant but harmless activity, perhaps moderately useful in promoting the patient's compliance with a medication regime. Family therapists who want to make a place for their model in such a system must share the responsibility for treatment with the rest of the team and avoid, whatever they believe, taking the overt position that the family is the real patient and the symptoms of the patient are only a representation of family pathology. It is far better to demonstrate the effectiveness of family interventions on a practical level and let other professionals conclude what they may. "True believers," however, may be unable to be this flexible, placing themselves in a power struggle with the rest of the staff, and tending to forget the important therapeutic principle of joining a system where it is. When practicing family therapy such therapists would probably avoid having an immediate "showdown" with a family, but somehow they feel compelled to do so with their work systems. For example, some true believers loudly oppose the use of medication, deny the need ever to talk with patients individually, or object to any action that they believe would reinforce the idea that there is a patient within the family. These positions are guaranteed to alienate all other members of the team not trained in family therapy, and even some who are.

This is not to say that family therapists always cause the interstaff struggles and resistances to family therapy. Even when family therapists are not true believers and have taken care to enter the treatment system cautiously, persistent inattention to family issues can eventually drive them to a sort of situational paranoia in which they begin to see the medical model as a plot on the part of the power structure to maintain control over the care-giving system. For instance, an oversight by the supervising physician or the agency supervisor in not considering the data from the family evaluation when formulating the overall treatment strategy can become a major affront to the aspiring family therapist's sense of worth as a member of the staff. Several such oversights in a row may lead to a bad case of therapist fatigue and a sense of alienation from the rest of the staff. Unless they can have an impact on attitudes and policies in these situations, therapists who are trying to see families are likely to either give up or find another system in which to practice.

Even when family therapy is an accepted part of the services given by an agency or institution, conflict between the family therapist and the rest of the staff can occur if those on the staff not trained in family therapy try to dictate the goals and methods of the family therapy part of the treatment plan. For example, their staff member may overidentify with the individual patient and urge the family therapist to make interventions in the family which would protect the patient from criticism by his/her family, regardless of what this would do to the long-term progress of the patient or the family. In such situations family therapists can become triangulated between families and other staff, so that they find themselves defending family members from the real or imagined assaults of staff members, or getting into pointless struggles with the rest of the team over the "real" goals of therapy. They may begin to overreact to remarks of other staff members. For instance, a colleague recently was unduly irritated when a nurse remarked that a patient's husband was "a real bastard" because he became angry at the patient when she had anxiety attacks, forgetting that this particular nurse had not had an opportunity to see the role this woman's symptom played in punishing her husband for alleged neglect and binding him to her through her weakness.

Administrative resistance, or the nuisance factor

Another major source of institutional resistance to family therapy is usually found primarily among administrators, and can be said to be caused by its "nuisance factor." Family therapy is a nuisance in all systems, but particularly in psychiatric or mental health systems accustomed to seeing patients individually. Administrators are confronted with hitherto unknown problems. Who gets a chart? Who must have a physical? Who must have a mental status exam? Who gets a diagnosis? Who *is* the patient? In other words, family therapy is a nuisance for administrators because it doesn't fit neatly with the practices and procedures which have been designed for the individual patient.

Take the relatively simple matters of registering patients and charting their progress. This is usually done by assigning a patient a number and establishing a chart with that person's name and number on it. What should be done if there are more family members to be seen than the member who originally presented with symptoms? Should each person become a "case" with a separate number, or should a family chart be established? If separate charts are established for each family member, can it be insured that copies of documents common to all family members are included in all the charts? The Xerox budget will skyrocket. Must already overworked clinicians write a separate note for each family member? Notes will get shorter or the families they see will get smaller. If family charts are established, other problems are presented. What if more than one family member requires individualized treatments such as medication or hospital admission? If a husband and wife divorce, what becomes of their chart; can each have access to it and/or use it against the other? Is there a way of insuring confidentiality between family members in such battles? If one number is given to the whole family with letters signifying which member has which chart, how can family charting be integrated with a computerized system programmed to handle one member at a time and not the occasional case number with tagalong letters? Family therapy is also a nuisance for administrators in terms of billing procedures. Computers are unaccustomed to more than one number per case and some are therefore given to sending bills to random members of the family, and may even charge every member of the family for a given visit.

Family therapy is also a nuisance because its practice makes unusual and expensive demands of systems. Family therapists require larger offices and interviewing rooms. They require greater flexibility in arranging appointments which are possible for all family members, thereby increasing the hours the agency or clinic is required to be open. It's expensive and inconvenient to keep clinics open at night. It is also inconvenient for therapists who would rather spend their evenings with their own families. Furthermore, the clinic statistics often look worse when clinicians do family therapy because the needs of multiple family members result in more staff time per case and thus fewer cases. While there is some evidence that family therapy can shorten or even avoid the necessity of hospitalization, this may not always be viewed as an advantage by administrators who must keep a full census to insure the economic survival of hospitals.

The training requirements of family therapists also make expensive demands upon the system. While discussing a family session is more useful than having no supervision at all, videotapes or live supervision are far superior. Videotaped demonstrations by experienced therapists allow beginners to view the family process without the anxiety of having to conduct the therapy, while observing their own videotapes with supervisors allows for accelerated learning both about families and about therapeutic interventions. Live supervision creates an even more accelerated learning process since beginners can get immediate feedback from their supervisors and see the effects of their revised interventions. However, videotape equipment is expensive to install and maintain, and live supervision is expensive in terms of supervisory time. Administrators are not always sure that the costs don't outweigh the benefits.

Resistances of larger systems

In our society almost all institutions and agencies have multiple sources of funding, many of which exercise control over how the funds are spent. Funds supplied by state and federal sources come with instructions on how the money is to be spent, and third-party payers are specific about which services qualify for reimbursement and which do not. Third-party payers are accustomed to paying for treatment for individual patients. They have their own rules and regulations and most of them don't have room for the idea of the family as the patient. Family therapy presents reimbursement problems unless there is a family member with a clear-cut disorder which can be labeled under the current psychiatric nosology. Someone in the family must bear a label for a condition which is reimbursable under the current system. This necessity is distasteful to many family therapists from an ideological point of view and can undermine the course of treatment by unnecessarily prolonging a focus on one particular family member.

Third-party payers may create resistance to family therapy in families and institutions by making the process of getting reimbursed more difficult. For example, one insurance company actually responded to a patient's claim for reimbursement for family therapy by saying that family therapy would be considered a reimbursable treatment only if everyone in the family was sick with a separate, reimbursable psychiatric disorder which could be labeled and justified according to DSM-III criteria. In this particular case, the husband of a depressed woman also would have had to be labeled depressed or as having some other definable disorder in order for the family to qualify for ongoing insurance coverage. Hours of extra paperwork by the therapist and the hospital system finally convinced this particular insurance company that when certain chronic symptoms are associated with specific relational difficulties, family therapy is in order and should be reimbursed. This, however, was one of only many battles, most of which are lost. For instance, if no one person contains a symptom cluster, as is often true with couples presenting with marital difficulties, obtaining a third-party payment is difficult if not impossible. Families, couples, and therapists may prefer to try to resolve problems individually rather than dealing directly with these systems resistances.

Larger systems make other demands on the time of all therapists by requiring a bewildering array of reports, summaries, treatment plans, and other forms of paperwork. The requirement that family therapists fill out such forms or compose such summaries separately for each member of a family puts an extra burden on practicing family therapists and discourages many therapists from using a family approach. The magic of Xerox helps with some but not all of these tasks.

Special resistances caused by welfare and justice systems

Some larger systems make family therapy difficult because they place therapists in the position of both therapist and policeman. Caseworkers and probation officers are sometimes asked to do family therapy in the field while simultaneously playing a role in which they must hold a threat over the family's head that their income may be withdrawn or one or more family members will be placed in a foster home or institution. These workers have power over the fate of family members in a way that those working in mental health settings do not. Families are understandably hesitant to admit a potentially threatening professional into their confidence. They really would have to be crazy to welcome such an intrusion into their lives. This is not to say that such professionals cannot be helpful, but only that such workers will find it necessary to master all the resistances inherent in any change process plus the resistances generated by the complication of their dual role.

Whether it is possible for workers who represent authority also to establish therapeutic relationships with families represents a thorny question. The answer usually is a very qualified "Yes, if." Such therapists can be effective if the family is motivated; if there are support systems the worker can mobilize to help (such as foster grandparents to help overwhelmed mothers, recreation programs for bored adolescents, etc.); if case loads are small enough for the workers to have frequent contact with the families in their care; and particularly "yes, if" the workers can manage to demonstrate to families that they genuinely care about the needs of families and genuinely care about what happens to family members. If such family workers can communicate this caring to family members despite the coercive nature of their roles and the family's negative view of the authority or agency they represent it is possible to do effective family therapy.

Most representatives of large public agencies, however, are saddled with large case loads and are particularly vulnerable to the demands made by ever changing bureaucratic structures. In addition, they often must work in the field, which means trying to conduct family sessions in people's homes, frequently in the midst of the chaos and confusion of TVs blaring, neighborhood children coming and going, and the telephone ringing. It's a far cry from the sanctity of a session in a psychiatric clinic.

Considering the difficulties of conducting court-ordered or agency-decreed family therapy, it is no wonder that some resistance to doing family therapy is found in the therapists themselves. Conducting any kind of therapy under these conditions must seem rather like trying to slay a very large dragon with a very short sword. Caseworkers and probation officers ordered to do family therapy sometimes complain that their agency administrators have lost all touch with the problems of working in the field.

Resistances in families caused by inpatient psychiatric hospital systems

A particular kind of resistance is generated within families by current and/or past contact with inpatient psychiatric facilities. This is relevant since many of the severely disturbed patients seen in outpatient family therapy today have spent years going in and out of psychiatric hospitals with little change or improvement in either the patient's or the family's behavior. While this alone would be enough to discourage most families about the usefulness of professional help, many of these hospital experiences have seemed ineffective and even alienating to family members.

Most families hospitalize a member only after all else has failed. They do so in a crisis when feelings of guilt, anger, and hopelessness are high. They have no doubt been through a long period of attempting to cope with a patient whose behavior has been withdrawn, hostile, or irrational. When they come to the hospital they are usually already blaming themselves for the patient's illness or are at least suspecting they may have exacerbated it. The family, not just the patient, presents in crisis. To ignore the family or to use them only to gather a social history is to miss an opportunity to involve them in the patient's treatment and to communicate to the family that staff are concerned with their issues and problems.

Many chronic patients have been repeatedly hospitalized in state institutions located miles from the community in which the patient lives, further decreasing the chances of productive family involvement. Asking families to travel long distances to inconvenient locations is guaranteed to produce or exacerbate resistance. It guarantees that families will come infrequently and on weekends when treatment staff are unlikely to be present. When this is combined with the fact that years of treatment may not have produced much change, the stage is set for a failure to form treatment alliances between professionals and families.

Family resistance is also exacerbated by several more subtle processes inherent within such helping systems. For instance, on all inpatient units, staff have more contact with patients than with families and therefore tend to identify with patients and their problems. Since patients often become more upset when their families visit, staff tend to see families as destructive, intrusive, and disruptive of ward routine and the peace of the unit. Families also ask questions to which there are no answers and make staff feel incompetent. On the other hand, if families don't visit, staff tend to see them as uncaring and neglectful of patients. These evasive families may only be protecting themselves out of a fear of another negative experience with hospital staff, but it is unlikely that staff will see this healthy function of a family's behavior. In either case, staff tend to adopt a negative attitude toward family members which is projected in the way they treat them. Families very quickly get the idea that they are not welcome on the unit. This staff attitude, combined with the fact that families already feel guilty, overwhelmed, and useless, pretty much assures their distance from, if not actual hostility to, the treatment system.

If this process has happened many times with many hospital systems, families come to use hospitals only when they have "had it"; when they want to drop the patient and leave, using the hospitalization as a respite from the ongoing stress of living with a chronically dysfunctional and disruptive family member. If staff members now wish to involve such families in patients' treatments, they will have a hard row to hoe. These families have heard it all before. They have experienced the hope of quick remission being quashed, the sad experience of watching their relative deteriorate over time. They have been caught in conflicts between the patient and the staff of hospitals, and have learned to view any employee of a hospital with suspicion. They have seen the benefits of medication being overshadowed by the development of unpleasant and sometimes irreversible side effects. Often they have been the victims of the hostility of their ill relative. They are, in short, burned out. It would be unrealistic to expect a family to welcome an opportunity to rehash the patient's history, to re-experience the hostility of the staff, to hope for genuine change, unless this particular staff can prove they have something special to offer, and unless this particular staff can prove they will be more understanding of the family's needs.

Avoiding and overcoming common systems-based resistances

In all but those agencies and institutes which grew up specifically for the purpose of developing, testing, and nurturing family therapy, that is, those institutes organized by the founding fathers and mothers of family therapy, there is bound to be some system resistance to family therapy. Even with the unusual support that exists in the havens provided by family institutes, therapists still run the risk of occasionally contracting therapist fatigue, causing them to be resistant to particular families or to be resistant at particular times in their careers.

In order for resistance to family therapy to arise, someone in the system must represent support for at least the idea of family therapy. Just where in the system the support for family therapy is located determines a great deal about how resistance should be handled. A systems assessment is in order. The first part of this assessment must be of therapists themselves. Therapists who are untrained, or who are trained in an individual modality but are trying to learn family therapy, must ask themselves whether they really want to try a new modality that will no doubt be difficult. At least initially they must decide whether they can tolerate exposing their practice and how much they fear this exposure. They must decide whether they really have the time and energy. The second part of this assessment must determine the amount of supervisory and administrative support. Therapists should ascertain what their superiors think about the idea of family therapy and how much support supervisors and administrators are willing to give. If there is no direct source of support for family therapy within the system, therapists can look outside their own agency or institution for courses and workshops in family therapy, although this requires a truly independent spirit.

On the other hand, even if there is strong administrative support for family therapy, family therapists can expect to encounter some reservations by those senior clinicians not trained in family therapy, and perhaps some reluctance on the part of the financial officer to purchase the equipment needed for training and supervision. These more passive resistances can still be quite powerful in preventing successful family therapy, but they require different strategies of intervention. The rest of this chapter details some forms of resistances to family therapy residing in or engendered by helpers and helping systems, followed by suggested methods of coping with them.

Problem 1. Therapist-based resistance due to competence anxiety

There is no way to avoid this sort of resistance since it is inherent in the situation of beginning to learn a new method of conducting therapy. Everyone feels it during the beginning stages of learning anything and most therapists feel it periodically throughout their careers. The only question is how much you are going to let it interfere with your behavior. In family therapy training, competence anxiety is frequently complicated by the need to expose one's practice through videotape and live supervision, a process which can exacerbate any beginner's anxiety.

SUGGESTIONS

Seek Good Supervision. Therapists need support and understanding from supervisors or colleagues, particularly early in their careers. If beginners have a choice of supervisors, they should make that choice carefully. Sometimes people with a great deal of knowledge about families are essentially not very good at being warm and supportive, and some people who are warm and supportive don't really know very much about families. Not that supervisors must be gushy to be supportive, but rather they must be sensitive to the issues faced by beginning therapists. Ideally, beginning therapists should select supervisors who are both supportive and who have demonstrated ability. One way to judge the family skills of supervisors is to get permission to observe their practice, either live or on tape. Not only does this give beginning therapists a chance to see the approach of potential supervisors and to judge whether they are simpatico, but the mere fact that supervisors are willing to freely expose their own practice is a good sign. Such supervisors are more likely to be open in other ways as well.

If beginners must choose betwen a supervisor who is supportive versus one who is knowledgeable, they should make this choice by considering their own needs. If they know they tend to respond catastrophically to criticism and/or that they have little support elsewhere in their lives, then they must choose the supportive supervisor in order to survive. If they can grit their teeth and learn while they are uncomfortable, then beginners will probably gain much more from a knowledgeable, but critical mentor. In either case, beginners must choose someone they respect.

Learn to Use Supervision Wisely. If they do not have a free choice of supervisors, and even if they do, it is important that beginning therapists take responsibility for their own learning, and to some degree, responsibility for what happens in supervision. For instance, beginning family therapists may need to learn to be specific about the kind of support they need or can tolerate. It is sometimes easy for supervisors to forget how difficult it is to begin seeing families, or how threatening it is to expose one's practice to the scrutiny of another. Beginners must be willing to give supervisors feedback, or to ask questions when a suggestion doesn't make sense. If beginning therapists cannot challenge their supervisors, they will probably find themselves ignoring their supervision or sabotaging suggested interventions. To get true support from supervision, therapists must be willing to say, "That sounds like a good suggestion, but I don't think I can do it." Remember, no one expects beginning therapists to know what they are doing, least of all the supervisors to whom they expose their work. If therapists feel overwhelmed with the number of things to learn in supervision, they can ask their supervisors to help them focus on one or two important issues. If novices know, for example, that their first task is to learn to hold a focus in a family interview, they can ask to concentrate on that issue in supervision and temporarily stop worrying about following complicated transactional behavior patterns.

Arrange for Other Ongoing Supports. Braulio Montalvo once was heard to tell two overextended parents that "good parenting begins with each other," making the point that to care for children, parents must first nurture themselves. This is also true of therapists. For this reason, if experienced supervision is not available, beginning therapists should care for themselves by seeking support in other ways. Any health care delivery system or community referral agency usually contains several persons who are interested in family therapy but are isolated from each other. Family therapists who put some effort into organizing a study group, lunchtime case conference, or who take the initiative to spend time with each of these isolated persons discussing family therapy will find themselves rewarded with better morale, a valuable support system, and an increased number of referrals.

Confess. Speakers suffering from stage fright have sometimes been told to announce at the beginning of their speeches that they are paralyzed with anxiety. The philosophy behind this tactic is that once they have announced that they may completely fail to perform, their anxiety will be reduced greatly because they are relieved of the anxiety of covering up their anxiety. Beginners need not confess to families that they are anxious, but they can at least do so to themselves, their supervisors, and their peers whose opinions they value. Once they have exposed their anxiety, they don't have to be so concerned with covering it up and can concentrate more fully on the family in front of them or on what their supervisor is trying to teach them.

Problem 2. Clinician resistance due to therapist fatigue

Like other forms of systems-based resistance, therapist fatigue is usually projected outward so that it appears to reside in family systems. Families begin missing appointments, responding perhaps to small, unconscious messages sent by therapists. Families are amazingly sensitive to whether or not therapists really want to see them. In fact, one way to tell when therapists need vacations is when an unusually large number of their families begin to cancel appointments.

SUGGESTIONS

Consult with Colleagues. It is a good idea for therapists to talk over frustrations with colleagues whom they can trust to be reasonably objective and appreciative of the problem. Even if their colleagues have no good solutions for resolving a particular frustration, there is usually some relief inherent in verbalizing it (the old get-it-off-your-chest routine). In such discussions, it sometimes helps to ask other therapists what they do when they are worn out, or to ask for specific help in looking at the way one's time and energies are organized.

Review Videotapes. Since clinician-based resistance is often projected out onto the family, it can be helpful to review videotapes of recent interviews for some perspective on the problems which have developed in therapist–family interaction. Particularly resistant families may make their therapists unconsciously angry or impatient, draining therapeutic energies in the process. Therapists may be able to recognize that their own attitudes are less supportive than usual, that they are being more demanding of family members than is really warranted, or that they are just not behaving in their usual therapeutic way. Recognizing their own fatigue is often enough to free them up to do something about it, and thus gives them the ability to cure their own problems.

Change the Content or Pace of the Case Load. If therapists find themselves resisting their families consistently, sometimes it is a case of needing to rethink their own or their agency's policy on the numbers of cases therapists can manage. If therapists are seeing families rather than individuals, usually their overall case load must be smaller. On the other hand, sometimes it is the particular nature of the case load that is causing fatigue. For example, therapists carrying a heavy case load of families containing patients with chronic schizophrenia may be more vulnerable to therapist fatigue than a clinician with a well-rounded case load.

If certain families are producing therapist fatigue, it may be advisable to space their appointments out, leaving two or three weeks between appointments. This may or may not slow down the change process, but it certainly is better than therapists blowing the whole therapeutic relationship because they are overloaded. Sometimes, it is necessary for therapists to admit they cannot be all things to all people and that there are some families which are particularly unappealing to them. When a therapist does not like a family or feels a particular family stirs up his/her personal issues, his/her freedom to intervene is curtailed. If therapists cannot get a handle on their own resistance by any of the methods mentioned here or in Chapter 4, the most ethical action is to transfer the cases that are stimulating these reactions.

Problem 3. Systems resistances based on unfamiliarity with family therapy

As mentioned in the beginning of this chapter, nonfamily therapists have usually heard of family therapy but are not familiar with its underlying principles, and often assume it is a form of individual therapy carried on with several members of the family in the room.

In many cases, agencies and institutions decide to include family therapy in their services without a clear understanding of its theories and methods and then find themselves having to deal with a treatment modality and/or a staff member who simply doesn't fit in with standard agency practices. The type of resistance the system will express will depend on whether the family therapist is experienced elsewhere but new to this particular system, or whether a professional within the system is attempting to learn and implement a family therapy program.

SUGGESTIONS

Enter the System Carefully — through the Power Structure. If family therapists are coming from outside the system, they will encounter difficulties enough with established procedures and natural resistances to change without immediately taking on an entire agency, and attempting to convert it to their point of view. Obtaining the support of the administration is crucial. It will not guarantee success in getting others to "think family," but at least it will prevent a guaranteed failure. Administrative support gives family therapists a ticket of admission, a chance to prove the usefulness of this type of treatment. In entering such systems, family therapists should carefully choose what's realistic to accomplish and what will help to demonstrate the case for family therapy. Given the characteristics of the system, therapists may choose to take easy cases of relatively certain positive outcome, or the most difficult cases no one wants to treat.

Avoid Evangelism and Hopeless Power Struggles. Most family therapists must reconcile themselves to practicing cooperatively in settings which are and will be dominated by an individual model, whether it be a psychological model, a biological model, or both. After all, Charcot and Freud predated Jackson, Minuchin, and Bowen by almost a century.

In the struggle for recognition as a respectable treatment modality in traditional psychiatric circles, family therapists have taken some rather untenable stands about the etiology of psychopathology. There is no good, hard evidence that anyone's family can drive them literally crazy, although many of us certainly believe we have experiential evidence to the contrary. Current research into the etiology of psychopathology indicates there are probably strong biological factors in both schizophrenia and depression and, no matter how logical or distinct the role of the family seems in psychosomatic disorders, there are no epidemiological studies which offer any credible evidence of the role of the family in the etiology of these disorders. These arguments do not detract from the importance of family systems and family therapy. Even if it is eventually discovered that the etiology of certain mental conditions is completely genetic or biochemical, families would still be relevant to symptom maintenance, and the course or outcome of the illness. Credible evidence exists that families influence the *course* of schizophrenia and such evidence is probably forthcoming for depression. Further, evidence exists that family intervention is as effective as psychiatric hospitalization and has fewer negative after effects. There is, therefore, no point in arguing about the etiology of illness. Such arguments only alienate colleagues and further polarize an already polarized field.

Family therapists, should, above all, resist getting into power struggles over which theory is the most "right," whether they are dealing with strict adherents of psychodynamic theory or a collection of therapists trained in models ranging from psychodynamic to behavior modification. Such power struggles can ruin staff morale and undermine therapists' confidence in themselves and their practice. One of the authors had the unfortunate experience of being hired as a family therapist by an agency with a strict psychoanalytic orientation. Having come from one of those institutes organized around one of the founding fathers where family therapy was close to a religion, she breezily assumed the staff would be as excited about her new approach as she was. As she attempted to convert everyone to the family point of view, the staff responded by labeling her behavior as "disturbed," that is, as a manifestation of her problems separating from her former agency, and she was treated with condescension. Needless to say, she separated from that agency as soon as possible, having learned something about the potentially negative effects of evangelism.

Prove to Be Helpful and of Good Will. If a system does not know about family therapy and its potential benefits, it will not use it productively. Family therapists have to go the extra mile to prove that there is a place for family therapy within the system and that it is in everyone's best interests to use it. In entering a system that was very skeptical, unknowledgeable, and hostile about family therapy, one of the authors placed the family therapy staff on 24-hour call to the emergency room. If anyone who had a family arrived with any sort of problem, she promised a family therapist would be available to deal with it. Such an offer was an imposition on a very small staff, and essentially unnecessary if the emergency room staff were only willing to refer families to family therapy. However, political and emotional issues in the system were blocking such referrals and it was clear that family therapists had to do something dramatic to prove themselves. Despite the fact that many reasonable family cases came in at convenient hours, the staff were not called. They *were* called for several nearly hopeless situations on Sundays and in the middle of the night, clearly more to test the offer than to refer cases. When the family therapists cheerfully responded to such calls, took the referrals seriously, and attempted to see these difficult cases, the midnight calls stopped and more reasonable referrals were made. Whenever a good referral was made, or whenever genuine improvement in difficult cases was accomplished, the family staff made a point of getting back to the referral source and giving them feedback. Gradually these skeptical professionals began to ask more family oriented questions in their assessments, to think more about family issues, and to use the family therapy staff. While families never became their major preoccupation, at least family therapy got a foot in the door.

Bring Up Family Issues at Every Opportunity. Family therapists, or those interested in beginning to do family therapy in a system that does not recognize its value, should look for opportunities to raise staff consciousness about families. Such therapists should attend rounds, team meetings, and case conferences and listen carefully for family issues. By raising questions about families and by exploring the potential impact of families on individual functioning, family therapists can begin to interest the rest of the staff in family issues and thus to gain additional support for doing this type of therapy. In this process, family therapists must ask nonhostile, nonthreatening questions, and present a possible alternative way of explaining a behavior, rather than suggesting a truth. For instance, initially it may be helpful to ask questions about the patient's current family relationships: Do family members come to see him/her? Are they supportive or critical? Are there other stresses in the family right now? Might the family be willing to come in? Initially, it might also be helpful to ask historical questions. Sometimes it is possible to demonstrate that the patient's symptoms have always worsened during times of high family stress such as after deaths of grandparents or when siblings left for college. In this way, staff may begin to see the relevance of family issues as a contributing force without having to sacrifice their basic theoretical orientations.

Don't Use Family Therapy Jargon. Institutional unfamiliarity with family therapy theory may be inadvertently exacerbated by family therapists who often find themselves in the position of having to educate their fellow clinicians to basic ideas such as "context." Basics may be boring, but family therapists who repeatedly launch complicated and sophisticated theoretical discussions may turn off their fellow practitioners and potential sources of referrals. While family therapists can be forgiven for occasionally engaging in this variation of psychobabble, they may leave their colleagues glassy-eyed and mistrustful. "Enmeshment," for example, is a term every family therapist understands but one which is difficult to explain to nonfamily therapists without the use of much gesticulating and "Well, I mean's," or even a videotape demonstration. It is much simpler to use more easily understood phrases such as "the family's shared anxiety," or describing the family as "so close that it's hard for them to have a difference of opinion, much less express it." Such explanations are more likely to encourage nonfamily therapists to notice events in terms of interactions and transactions. The truth is that while family therapy is quite difficult and complicated to learn to do, it is not difficult and complicated to understand. Simple explanations are often sufficient.

Make Analogies. Family therapists would be foolish to throw out all that has been learned about individual psychopathology and development or about other methods of influencing people therapeutically. Yet, rejection of all other theories and practices is often done when the establishment of the family systems point of view is treated as a political or semireligious crusade. There are plenty of connections between family therapy and other treatment modalities which can serve as useful bridges for engendering understanding and cooperation with other therapists.

Behavior therapists understand the principles of extinguishing certain behaviors while rewarding others, which is certainly a part of what goes on in family therapy. Colleagues with a behavioral orientation can see the family therapist as selectively rewarding some behaviors and punishing others once he/she is inside the family boundary. The family therapist's selective use of alignments and tasks to strengthen generational boundaries also can be viewed in behavioral terms. It is quite easy to explain this sort of therapy to behavior modification buffs without ever using the word "system."

With physicians, it is sometimes useful to make analogies which connect family systems issues to the myriad of regulatory systems in the human body. Doctors are familiar with the notion of systems, just not systems which go beyond the skin of one person. A simple analogy such as "I believe this patient's anxiety attacks are exacerbated by her husband's criticism, just like an ulcer is exacerbated by stress or spicy food," will go far to explain the family therapist's point of view.

Present Cases. It is important to take advantage of all opportunities to present case material to colleagues of different backgrounds. In such presentations, it is useful to demonstrate the role that families play in the maintenance of symptoms and/or in their exacerbation, since this point is less controversial than many others. If therapists can demonstrate, by outlining the sequence of events or by showing videotapes of family sessions, that when family anxiety is raised an exacerbation of symptomatic behavior in the patient results, they begin to make the case for family systems thinking. This is the first step toward gaining support for doing family work, and perhaps even convincing others to do it, too.

The strategic use of videotapes deserves a special note. If therapists are lucky enough to have videotape equipment, they should use it liberally to make their teaching points. It is important, however, that therapists not get carried away with their own fascination with family dynamics and their own brilliant interventions. Colleagues are more receptive to short, readily understandable demonstrations of family dynamics which can be easily related to symptom maintenance. To make an effective point, therapists should pick one aspect of a family's dynamics and demonstrate it dramatically and repeatedly throughout a presentation. For example, if therapists wish to show how family members avoid conflict by scapegoating the patient, they should show three clear examples of no more than 2 minutes' duration each, and then explain how this is related to symptom maintenance. Ruthless editing of videotapes is in order. If a sophisticated support network for the making and editing of videotapes is not available, therapists should carefully prepare for presentations by noting the numbers on the videotape playback machine which correspond to the exact segments demonstrating their points. Many otherwise good presentations have been ruined by therapists searching for the right material while their colleagues became bored, irritated, or confused about the point of the demonstration.

Avoid Discussions of the Therapist's Own Family. Another pitfall family therapists sometimes encounter when educating their colleagues about family therapy theory is in attempting to use their own personal families to illustrate certain points. While many family therapists are fascinated by their own family origins and those of their colleagues, it is less likely that other professionals will be similarly impressed. Family therapists have become comfortable with such discussions over the years of their own training so that they fail to recognize that many of their fellow clinicians find this sort of self-disclosure embarrassing or even boring. Also, these discussions often involve complicated multigenerational genealogical charts and equally complicated explanations. People who are not devoted to family therapy become impatient with such discussions and may reject future discussions of family theory.

Problem 4. Resistances caused by the nuisance factors

Resistances generated by nuisance factors, as has been mentioned, relate to space, records, billing, and the time it takes to genuinely include families in a patient's care. The administration's attitude toward family therapy as it is expressed by their policies on such issues will be reflected by all other parts of the helping system. If the administration supports family therapy, the problems caused by its special needs will be overcome; if the administration is merely nonsupportive, family therapy will be difficult to practice and easy to ignore; if the administration is hostile, family therapy will be impossible.

That part of the system which keeps medical records and bills patients can cause particular chaos and thus resistance in families. Families who receive staggering bills because every member of the family has been independently charged for each session are more likely to drop out immediately. So are families where one member must spend hours on the phone trying to straighten out his/her bill because the computer has issued bills to family members randomly, and the person in the billing department has never heard of family therapy and doesn't understand the problem. By the time the harried family member explains that for reasons of third-party payment, income tax, and personal sanity, a bill for a single patient is needed with a single diagnosis and a legible list of sessions, instead of three different bills, with three different family members' names, and three conflicting lists of dates on which sessions were held, he/she can easily decide that termination is the better part of valor.

SUGGESTIONS

Evaluate the Source and Level of Nuisance-Related Resistance in the System. It is important to determine if nuisance-related resistances exist because no one has recognized their importance, because resources don't exist, or because no one cares. Is the reason there is no room available which is large enough to see families in because no one has taken the time to think through a new policy to involve families, or because the powers that be don't care if family therapy is done or not? Is the fact that the intake forms that must be completed on patients contain no mention of family issues due to lack of awareness of family issues, lack of respect for their importance, or lack of knowledge of what to ask? Are these shortcomings caused by lack of support at a senior level, or a lack of follow-through by middle-level management? One doesn't have to be a student of family systems to understand what lack of support from senior administration means.

Get a Commitment from the Administration. Before family therapists take on any other part of the helping system, they must have a commitment from the administration that family therapy is considered an important part of the services offered by the agency or institution and that he, she, or they support its practice. The level of support may be negotiable; that is, the amount of financial or emotional support the administration can provide may vary from system to system, but there must be an agreement in principle that family therapy is valid. In general, if there is no support from administration, and no clear way to demonstrate the usefulness of family therapy to gain that support, it is the better part of valor to give up doing family therapy in this particular system. Therapists should either move to another system or do the therapy that their system will support. The alternative is probably ulcers, low self-esteem, and/or acute loneliness.

Befriend People in Important Places. In order to win over support for a point of view, it often helps to make friends in various parts of the system and then make requests for assistance when problems arise. This is sometimes easier said than done because often it seems every part of the system has combined to make family therapy difficult. In the earlier example of family therapists putting themselves on call to the emergency room, the good will generated by that policy made it possible not only to get referrals, but to get emergency support for difficult cases. Whatever policies exist, it is the informal relationships and human contact that provides the oil which makes the system operate easily. Family therapists may get away with being high-handed, inconsiderate, or condescending to people lower in the hierarchy at a given moment, but in the long run, passive or active resistance from people who have been treated badly will work against them and the families they are attempting to help. It's an old and well-known tale that nurses on an inpatient unit are unlikely to awake unnecessarily on-call residents who have treated them as respected peers, while residents who have been obnoxious will invariably be disturbed at 3:00 A.M. for something the nursing staff could have handled easily on their own. Likewise, if family therapists have taken the trouble to make friends with line nursing staff, they will be more likely to be told about a family's Sunday visit that revealed some important family misunderstandings and resistances rather than having them explode in their faces. The family therapist who has dealt cheerfully with the billing department, helping to straighten out a problem bill may find that variations of rigid procedures can be arranged, even to the extent of having the billing people come to the therapist's office to discuss a problem with a family.

Visit the Gatekeepers Often. Conversations with the intake worker(s) or the chief resident, nurse, supervisor, or supervising physician in the intake unit allows for the sort of gentle probing and information sharing which was advocated in the earlier section of this chapter. Attending the staffings of the intake unit is an excellent way to educate staff as to what kinds of cases could benefit from family therapy, and what kinds of questions generate information about the relationship between the presenting problems and the patient's family. Furthermore, such conversations serve to keep the family therapist visible and family therapy on people's minds.

Volunteer to Revise Forms. All institutions design forms to insure that the information they think is necessary is gathered in a coherent form. Schools, courts, hospitals, and social agencies generally have designed their intake and treatment systems around individuals. For example, in one large acute care psychiatric hospital, the questions on the intake form designed to elicit information about family issues have been reduced to a simple block to be checked "Yes" or "No" in response to the question "Does the patient have family problems?" One can easily imagine that a busy clinician would simply check the box and not ask for details. The best way for family therapists to insure that family issues are included is to actually include them themselves, that is, to design questions which will elicit the kind of information regarding the context in which the patient's symptoms or problems appeared, and this in turn will stimulate the discussion of these issues. This almost automatically increases referrals for family therapy.

Send Memos. Memos are a system's formal method of communicating between subsystems. They are extremely useful for reminding various other subsystems that family therapy is alive and well at Extension 2389. They are also useful in bringing problems to the attention of the administration in a logical manner which is difficult to ignore. Perhaps the most underused function of memos, however, is for officially thanking various people for their help. Whether it be a secretary who made sure the family therapist was scheduled to use a room, a billing clerk who treated a family's complaint with tact, or an on-call physician who took the trouble to let the family therapist know that a family member dropped into the emergency room asking for medication, this can be a useful technique. Everyone complains when things go wrong. Few people compliment when things go right. If family therapists send memos, especially with copies to relevant supervisors, they can often be assured of future help and cooperation.

Problem 5. Resistances generated by the turf issue

The turf issues described in the early part of this chapter are likely to be caused by a lack of knowledge of the potential benefits of collaboration. Family therapy can and should be combined with other forms of psychotherapy and pharmacotherapy. In institutions which stress an individually oriented psychodynamic or biological approach to treatment, family therapy can usually be accepted at least as a method of securing the help of the patient's family in urging the patient to comply with treatment recommendations. If family therapists have serious reservations about the use of medication or individual contacts with patients then they ought not to work in hospitals or agencies where medication is prescribed or patients are seen in individual psychotherapy, or they will find themselves involved in power struggles with prescribing physicians which will be detrimental to patients and families.

Unless there is good will on both sides, the possible damage to the progress of treatment associated with toxic triangles between patients and different members of the treatment team is considerable. Such triangles occur mostly when the power structure supports some form of individual therapy as the treatment of choice with family intervention being regarded as a poor relation. In such systems, family sessions can be seen as disruptive, complicating the therapeutic alliance or the transference. The needs of patients are primary, even if other members of the patients' families have important conflicting needs. Without a family perspective, it is not easy to see that a temporary focus on their families' issues may be a short-term problem for patients, but better for them in the long run. This basic difference of perspective gets fought out in the areas of priorities, decisions, and who has the right to make them.

SUGGESTIONS

Keep the Hierarchy Sorted Out. Everyone is sensitive to having areas he/she considers his/her responsibility and area of expertise muscled in on by other members of the staff, particularly those in junior positions. Since family therapists are often not senior members of the treatment team, they should be sensitive to the power structure, and respectful of the boundaries of each team member's area of concern. There are bound to be areas in which responsibilities and interests of team members overlap, but family therapists should be particularly aware of and sensitive to these boundary and turf issues, and work to make their points without stepping on too many toes.

Define Treatment Goals and Methods. Very often the goals of various members of the treatment team may be the same but their methods are not. One way to avoid turf issues is for each person involved in the patient's treatment to contribute to the list of treatment goals, and for all members of the team to be aware of how each other's methods are contributing to reaching those goals. Open communication and respect among team members for what each one contributes is the key in making this technique work.

If All Else Fails, Confront Triangles. Family therapists are in the best position to diagnose unhealthy triangles because they are their own turf; that is, they have been trained to consider these systems and should take responsibility for being aware of them. This isn't easy, of course, since they, too, are emotionally involved. Nevertheless, they should attempt to be aware of when they are caught in triangles and to intervene by meeting directly with the member or members of the team with whom they see themselves in conflict. If a resident has been assigned to do family therapy, and a social worker undercuts her by meeting with the family informally during visiting hours, it is far better for her to deal directly with the social worker than to go to the ward chief to be rescued. In the long run the resolution of such conflicts is more important than winning a battle.

Problem 6. Special resistances produced by inpatient units

The resistances produced in families by staffs who either ignore them or are hostile because they have overidentified with the patient can be avoided or dispelled in a number of ways. While the resistances engendered by helping systems differ according to the characteristics of the system, it is hoped that some of the suggestions here can be applied to other settings, or at least generate a way of thinking about overcoming the impact of systems based resistances in general.

SUGGESTIONS

Establish Contact with the Family Immediately. As soon as patients are hospitalized, family therapists should establish contact with their families, suggesting they come in for a session without the patient. In addition to a focus on the patient's needs and problems, this session should include a focus on the family feelings about the patient and the situation. If a social history must be gathered, particular care should be taken to avoid transmitting the implication that the family's behavior has contributed to the patient's illness. If staff even unwittingly blame the family, the family will naturally avoid contact with staff. In early sessions, therefore, family therapists should take care to be supportive and to attend to the needs of family members, not just those of the patient. This includes helping the family to deal with their discouragement about the failure of helping systems to "cure" their relative, as well as dealing with the family's own anger, guilt, and sadness.

Be the Family's Representative to the Staff. It is important to help the inpatient staff to understand families. If staff are made aware of the difficulties the family has encountered with the patient, and reminded that the family's intrusiveness is a sign of concern or that their unavailability is a defense against despair, staff will be more sympathetic and project fewer hostile feelings on the patient's family. Also, therapists can report to family members what other members of the team are doing to help the patient, and why staff are making various treatment decisions. The family therapist can become the living link between the hospital and family systems.

Work to Move the System to a Family Perspective. The real goal of family therapists within hospital systems is usually not just to be allowed to do family therapy, or to get referrals of families, but to move the health care delivery system or community referral system toward a family model of health care delivery, that is, the inclusion of the family into the way the system treats the patient/client from the very beginning to the very end of treatment. In such a system, questions about family involvement and availability would be included in the first screening call so that family members learn to assume they will be included in the patient's treatment. In the assessment phase family members would be included in the assessment itself and in the decision making about the patient's treatment, rather than being asked to wait outside the interviewing room. In the case of inpatient units or group living agencies, visiting and appointment hours would be geared to promote frequent visiting and frequent family sessions. While family sessions might not include a member who is psychotic, early inclusion of sessions for other family members would keep them involved with the patient rather than encouraging them to drop the problem at the hospital and try to forget about it. To encourage a family model of health care, family therapists should consistently push to see that families are considered in every part of a patient's treatment and in every decision about treatment resources.

Problem 7. Resistances produced by court-ordered therapy

The imposition of forced therapy upon a family always sets up a situation in which extreme resistance can be expected. Therapists encounter court-ordered therapy primarily in two ways: They may simply be a therapist to whom a family has been sent by the legal system, or, they may actually be employed by or represent the legal system in some way. (This second type will be addressed in problem 8.) Therapists to whom the family has been sent can to some degree disassociate themselves from the court and proceed as they would in any other case. The separation is not entirely possible as the family members will be aware that the therapist will be asked for progress reports, but some boundary between therapist and authority can be established.

SUGGESTIONS

Make the Situation Explicit. When therapy is court ordered, it is best to state openly what everyone knows, that the family has come to therapy primarily because the judge ordered it. Therapists can then communicate that they understand that the family resents having to be there. This is a variation of the standard elicitation of overt resistance to avoid covert resistance. After some discussion of the feelings family members have about the coercive nature of the referral, therapists can restore the family's sense of control and responsibility by pointing out that they can, in fact, refuse the therapy and accept the consequences. While the consequences are usually serious enough to mean that this is not a desirable choice, it should be made clear that refusal is an option or they will continue to resist the therapist at every turn.

Negotiate an Explicit Contract. The problem in court-ordered therapy is to establish treatment contracts in which families retain some control while being realistic about the need to meet the court's demands as well. It is crucial to transfer some sense of responsibility for the outcome of therapy back to the family, or the therapist will be viewed as an arm of the court and resistance will be exacerbated. For instance, a therapist may say, "I have to write a letter to the court saying you are coming and working in therapy; but you must make a decision about what you want to work on and what you want to do with the sessions."

Because court-ordered therapy challenges a family's autonomy and sense of being in control, it is necessary to be very clear about the boundaries of therapy, the degree to which the court will be involved, and the type of reports that will be filed. Therapists should not exacerbate a family's sense of loss of control by being vague about what they will or won't do, what they will or won't offer, and what they will or won't report. The family must have the ability to give informed consent as to whether this whole process is worth their while.

It sometimes increases the family's sense of control to make it clear that reports given to other agencies will first be shared with the family. This does not mean that the family is necessarily asked to participate in writing such reports, although in cases where families are compliant and are making progress, inclusion in the process of writing the report would be a good way of reinforcing changes which have been made.

Avoid Overinvolvement in the Outcome. Most therapists are in the business because they like people and like to help. It is easy for therapists to become aligned with families facing difficult social and legal problems. Once this happens, the job of making tough decisions about whether real change has been achieved becomes even tougher. One of our students was assigned to see a couple whose infant daughter had been taken into protective custody after sustaining injuries during her parents' violent daily fights. The couple were at first resentful, hostile, and threatening toward the therapist but compliant in appearing for their sessions. In their relationship they were each so unsure of themselves and of the other's love that they argued violently each time one of them went out without the other. Neither would accept employment as it would mean long hours spent away from the other in the company of people of the opposite sex which was intolerable to both. Over the months, this couple became more friendly to the therapist. When they described their own difficult childhoods, it was easy for the therapist to begin to be sympathetic. Over time, they succeeded in stopping their violent fighting, which was usually initiated over issues of infidelity. Our student was quite proud that the couple had stopped fighting and prepared a report documenting their achievement. However, there was no evidence that the couple had made changes which would allow them to function as two autonomous adults responsible for the care of an infant. They had not attained a degree of maturity which would allow them to trust each other out of each other's sight, nor had they developed a social network to give them the necessary support and guidance they would need to take over the care of their daughter. Although the student wanted to write a good report for the court because he liked the couple and felt they were trying, he knew he could not say they were ready to care for a baby since he had no evidence to that effect. Reluctuantly, and to the couple's dismay he sided with the court's recommendation to not return the child at that time and to involve a parenting center which could provide a network of support on a daily basis.

Educate the Court about What Is Possible in Family Therapy. Family therapy holds so much promise to agencies used to considering the context of events that it may implicitly promise more than it can deliver. It is not possible to take a family which has been undermined from the beginning by poverty, crime, drugs, or whatever and turn it into a middle-class "haven in a heartless world." The child-abusing family needs more than crisis-oriented family therapy, it needs ongoing support and long-term help. Judges and other authorities may need to be educated as to the potential benefits and limitations of any kind of therapy, but particularly family therapy.

Problem 8. Resistances produced by actually representing authority

In these cases, the therapist/social worker/probation officer is directly associated with the court and in some way in a position to make direct recommendations to the court. In these cases, therapists cannot disassociate themselves from the source of the intrusive authority and must find a way to be helpful while still retaining authority. The family members know that a member could be sent to a correctional institution, or a child to a foster home, or not returned from a foster home, depending on the direct recommendations of the officer/therapist. These therapists must wear two hats, one white and one black. It is a very difficult trick to learn to switch hats at a moment's notice, although many welfare workers and probation officers become quite skilled at it. With their white hat on, they are consultants to families, standing as an equal in the power hierarchy, in fact, always being certain they do not overpower the parents lest these parents lose their needed leverage with their children. With their black hat on, however, these therapists represent society's power which supersedes that of the parents.

SUGGESTIONS

Define the Situation as a Crisis. Too often families which are ordered into therapy by society's representatives have adopted an attitude and a life-style in which events which would shake most families have become routine. Such routines may include arguments in which members assault each other, or in which members disappear for days at a time. Even the intrusion of social agencies has become routine. In order to generate any motivation, the situation has to be redefined into a crisis situation in which family members are expected to take some action. People are more likely to intervene if they see a situation as dangerous than if it is just more of the same. Redefining a situation as a crisis can be made more difficult if either the family has a long history of producing delinquent members or if they live in a neighborhood where most families share the chaotic life-style. For example, a probation officer asked a family therapy consultant what he could do for the youngest of 10 children in a family in which all the older siblings had been in and out of correctional and treatment facilities with no alteration in their antisocial behavior. Defining this child's behavior as an emergency would have no chance of altering the family's behavior since they were beyond emergencies. Nevertheless, the technique may work with less chronic patterns.

Make Concrete Suggestions. Just as they do in any crisis situation, therapists should take charge, provide structure, and make concrete suggestions as to what family members can do to change things. These families cannot use reflective, supportive, or insight-oriented family therapy. What is needed is imaginative thinking, drawing on the existing or potential support networks the family has at their disposal. For example, in a family which had raised several children successfully but whose youngest son was flirting with delinquency and drug use, the probation officer realized that the parents' authority had been lessened by degenerative illnesses. He declared the situation a crisis and suggested they summon their grown children to come and help them. The situation was resolved by having one of the boy's adult brothers take him back to his home in Arizona to remove him from his peer group, and to provide a source of support and guidance for the remaining years it would take him to mature.

Reinforce the Power Structure. It is very important when intervening with families in court-ordered therapy to try to put the power of the court behind those individuals in the family who seem most capable of exercising authority, or who should be exercising authority but aren't. For example, the mother in a family which included a 19-year-old son who was drinking and abusing drugs was trying to establish control but was clearly overwhelmed by her son's sheer size. Several phone calls by the therapist to this boy's passively resistant father were unsuccessful in getting him to come to therapy sessions. It was only when the therapist threw the weight of his own power and that of the court behind the strong message to the father that he was the only person who could save his son that the father was finally mobilized to action. He came with his wife to a therapy session during which they worked out a set of rules which the father was willing to support. Of course after years of passively watching his wife manage the children, he was not immediately effective, but it was a start.

Problem 9. Resistances produced by working in the field

Most court-ordered therapy done by welfare workers and probation officers takes place in their clients' homes. When family therapy must be conducted on the family's own turf, there are usually many uncontrollable intrusions into sessions in the form of small children, animals, TV and radio, neighbors, etc., which can be used by family members as resistances to therapy. These interruptions, plus the question of the therapist's personal safety, also produce resistance to therapy within the workers themselves.

SUGGESTIONS

Establish Boundaries Early. Realistically one cannot come into a family's home and take over without some social interaction, and all therapy sessions ought to include some basic social interaction as a sign of respect and friendliness. However, therapy is never a social situation. A home setting can distract people from the serious purpose of the meeting. It is very important that the therapist establish the boundaries early. No, it is not okay if the TV or radio is on or Johnny from next door is over playing. All family members participating in therapy should be in the room.

Set Time Limits. Again, the structure of sessions held in the office is often set by the habits of a particular agency. Most sessions are either a half-hour, an hour, or whatever time period is necessary for the usual business to take place. In the home there is no such structure. Sessions can be anywhere from 10 minutes to several hours in duration, if therapists don't announce what their expectations are. Of course, in time of crisis one does what one has to do, but for ongoing therapy, a time limit should be set. One of the authors was once involved in what turned out to be marathon therapy in the home of a 14-year-old boy who refused to leave his home. She failed to establish early her expectations about the length of the session, and as the family was large and everyone wanted his/her say, the session ran well over 3 hours. Needless to say, she was exhausted at its completion and hadn't had the energy to make effective interventions for the last hour.

Summary

This chapter has been concerned with those resistances which, although they are frequently projected out on families actually reside either in therapists or the helping systems in which they work, or are produced by these helping systems but are expressed by families. Resistances residing in therapists include those produced in beginners by competence anxiety or ambivalence about the efficacy of family therapy, and those produced by therapist fatigue in both beginners and experienced therapists. Resistances residing in agencies and institutions include those produced by the unfamiliarity of senior staff with the underlying principles of family therapy, institutional *diablos conocidos,* those habitual procedures which tend to perpetuate old attitudes and practices, and those resistances produced by irritation with the evangelism of family therapy "true believers." Institutional resistances are also caused by the nuisance factor, that is, all those billing and record-keeping problems engendered by having more than one patient per case, plus the need for bigger offices and flexible hours. Other resistances are caused by the larger systems which influence what type of therapy is financially viable. Special resistances are caused by the authoritative position of those therapists who practice in welfare and justice systems. Finally, resistances within families can be produced by inpatient units who neglect or are overtly hostile to family members.

Bibliography

Ackerman, N. W. Family psychotherapy and psychoanalysis: Implications of difference. In N. W. Ackerman (Ed.), *Family process.* New York: Basic Books, 1970, pp. 5–18.

Aponte, H. J., & Van Deusen, J. M. Structural family therapy. In A. S. Gurman & D. P. Kniskern (Eds.), *Handbook of family therapy.* New York: Brunner/Mazel, 1981, pp. 310–360.

Ard, B. Reality, reframing and resistance in therapy: Interview with P. Watzlawick. *AAMFT Family Therapy News,* January 1982, *13,* 1.

Barker, P. *Basic family therapy.* Baltimore: University Park Press, 1981.

Bateson, G., Jackson, D., Haley, J., & Weakland, J. Toward a theory of schizophrenia. *Behavioral Science,* 1956, *1,* 251–264.

Beck, A., Rush, A. J., Shaw, B., & Emery, G. *Cognitive therapy of depression.* New York: Guilford Press, 1979.

Boszormenyi-Nagy, I., & Spark, G. *Invisible loyalties.* New York: Harper & Row, 1973.

Boszormenyi-Nagy, I., & Ulrich, D. N. Contextual family therapy. In A. S. Gurman & D. P. Kniskern (Eds.), *Handbook of family therapy.* New York: Brunner/Mazel, 1981, pp. 159–186.

Bowen, M. *Family therapy in clinical practice.* New York: Jason Aronson, 1978.

Brehm, J. W. *Response to loss of freedom: A theory of psychological resistance.* Morristown, N.J.: General Learning Press, 1972.

Burke, J. D., White, H. S., & Havens, L. L. Which short-term therapy? *Archives of General Psychiatry,* 1979, *36,* 177–186.

Carter, E. A., & McGoldrick, M. (Eds.). *The family life cycle: A framework for family therapy.* New York: Gardner Press, 1980.

D'Alessio, G. The concurrent use of behavior modification and psychotherapy. *Psychotherapy: Theory, Research and Practice,* 1968, *5*(3), 154–159.

Davanloo, H. (Ed.). *Short-term dynamic psychotherapy.* New York: Jason Aronson, 1980.

Dell, P. J. Beyond homeostasis: Toward a concept of coherence. *Family Process,* 1982, *21*(1), 21–41.

de Shazer, S. *The death of resistance.* Unpublished manuscript, 1980.

de Shazer, S. *Patterns of brief family therapy: An ecosystemic approach.* New York: Guilford Press, 1982.

Dicks, H. V. *Marital tensions: Clinical studies towards a psychological theory of interaction.* London: Routledge & Kegan Paul, 1967.

Epstein, N. B., & Bishop, D. S. Problem-centered systems therapy of the family. In A. S. Gurman & D. P. Kniskern (Eds.), *Handbook of family therapy.* New York: Brunner/Mazel, 1981, pp. 444–482. (a)

Epstein, N. B., & Bishop, D. S. Problem-centered systems family therapy. *Journal of Marital and Family Therapy,* 1981, *7*(1), 23–32. (b)

Epstein, N. B., Bishop, D. S., & Levin, S. The McMaster model of family functioning. *Journal of Marriage and Family Counseling,* 1978, *4,* 19–31.

Erickson, M. H. Indirect hypnotic therapy of a bedwetting couple. *Journal of Clinical and Experimental Hypnosis,* 1954, *2,* 171–174.

Ferenczi, S. *Further contributions to the theory and technique of psychoanalysis.* London: Hogarth Press, 1950.

Fogarty, R. F. Systems concepts and the dimensions of self. In P. J. Guerin (Ed.), *Family therapy: Theory and practice.* New York: Gardner Press, 1976, pp. 144–153.

Forrest, T. Treatment of the father in family therapy. *Family Process,* 1969, *8*(1), 106–108.

Framo, J. L. The integration of marital therapy with sessions with family of origin. In A. S. Gurman & D. P. Kniskern (Eds.), *Handbook of family therapy.* New York: Brunner/Mazel, 1981, pp. 133–158.

Frank, J. *Persuasion and healing.* Baltimore: The John Hopkins University Press, 1961.

Frankenstein, R. Agency and client resistance. *Social Casework,* January 1982, 24–28.

Freud, S. *A general introduction to psychoanalysis.* New York: Washington Square Press, 1952. (Originally published, 1900.)

Friedman, E. H. The birthday party: An experiment in obtaining change in one's own extended family. *Family Process,* 1971, *10*(3), 345–359.

Fromm-Reichmann, F. *Principles of intensive psychotherapy.* Chicago: University of Chicago Press, 1950.

Garfield, S. L. Research on client variables in psychotherapy. In S. L. Garfield & A. E. Bergin (Eds.), *Handbook of psychotherapy and behavior change* (2nd ed.). New York: Wiley, 1971, pp. 271–298.

Greenson, R. R. *The technique and practice of psychoanalysis.* New York: International Universities Press, 1967.

Guerin, P. J. The use of the arts in family therapy: I never sang for my father. In P. J. Guerin (Ed.), *Family therapy: Theory and practice.* New York: Gardner Press, 1976, pp. 480–500.

Guerin, P. J., & Pendagast, E. G. Evaluation of family system and genogram. In P. J. Guerin (Ed.), *Family therapy: Theory and practice.* New York: Gardner, 1976, pp. 450–464.

Gurman, A. S., & Kniskern, D. P. (Eds.). *Handbook of family therapy.* New York: Brunner/Mazel, 1981.

Hadley, T., Jacob, T., Milliones, J., Caplan, J., & Spitz, D. The relationship between family developmental crises and the appearance of symptoms in a family member. *Family Process,* 1974, *13*, 2.

Haley, J. *Uncommon therapy: The psychiatric techniques of Milton A. Erickson, M.D.* New York: W. W. Norton, 1973.

Haley, J. Why a mental health clinic should avoid family therapy. *Journal of Marriage and Family Counseling,* 1975, *1*(2), 3–13.

Haley, J. *Problem solving therapy.* San Francisco: Jossey-Bass, 1976.

Heath, T. Review of "On window shopping or being a non-customer" by L. Segal and P. Watzlawick. *The Underground Railroad,* 1981, *2*(3), 3.

Hersen, M. Resistance to direction in behavior therapy: Some comments. *Journal of Genetic Psychology,* 1971, *118*, 121–127.

Hersen, M. Limitations and problems in the clinical application of behavioral techniques in psychiatric settings. *Behavior Therapy,* 1979, *10*, 65–80.

Hoffer, E. *The ordeal of change.* New York: Harper & Row, 1963.

Hoffman, L. Deviation-amplifying processes in natural groups. In J. Haley (Ed.), *Changing families.* New York: Grune & Stratton, 1971, pp. 285–311.

Hoffman, L. *Foundations of family therapy.* New York: Basic Books, 1981.

Hofstadter, D. R. *Gödel, Escher, Bach: An eternal golden braid,* New York: Basic Books, 1979.

Hoyt, M. F., Henley, M. D., & Collins, B. E. Studies in forced compliance: Confluence of choice and consequences on attitude change. *Journal of Personality and Social Psychology,* 1972, *23*, 204–210.

Jackson, D. D. The study of the family. *Family Process,* 1965, *4*, 1–20.

Jacobson, N. S. Behavioral marital therapy. In A. S. Gurman & D. P. Kniskern (Eds.), *Handbook of family therapy.* New York: Brunner/Mazel, 1981, pp. 556–591.

Jacobson, N. S., & Margolin, G. *Marital therapy: strategies based on social learning and behavior exchange principles.* New York: Brunner/Mazel, 1979.

Jahn, D. L., & Lichstein, K. L. The resistive client: A neglected phenomenon in behavior therapy. *Behavior Modification,* 1980, *4*(3), 303–320.

Johnston, T. F. Hooking the involuntary family into treatment: Family therapy in a juvenile court setting. *Family Therapy,* 1974, *1,* 79–82.

Kanfer, F. H. Self-management methods. In F. H. Kanfer & A. P. Goldstein (Eds.), *Helping people change.* New York: Pergamon, 1975, pp. 309–355.

Kerr, M. E. Family systems theory and therapy. In A. S. Gurman & D. P. Kniskern (Eds.), *Handbook of family therapy.* Brunner/Mazel, 1981, pp. 226–266.

Kopel, S., & Arkowitz, H. The role of attribution and self-perception in behavior change: Implications for behavior therapy. *Genetic Psychology Monographs,* 1975, *92,* 175–212.

Lansky, M. R. On blame. *International Journal of Psychoanalytic Psychotherapy,* 1980, *8,* 429–460.

Lansky, M. R. Family psychotherapy in the hospital. In M. R. Lansky (Ed.), *Family therapy and major psychopathology.* New York: Grune & Stratton, 1981, pp. 395–414.

Larson, C. C., & Gilbertson, D. L. Reducing family resistance to therapy through a child management approach. *Social Casework,* December 1977, 620–623.

Liberman, R. P. Managing resistance to behavioral family therapy. In A. S. Gurman (Ed.), *Questions and answers in the practice of family therapy.* New York: Brunner/Mazel, 1981, pp. 186–194.

Luther, G., & Loev, I. Resistance in marital therapy. *Journal of Marital and Family Therapy,* 1981, *7*(4), 421–572.

Mahoney, M. J. *Cognition and behavior modification.* Cambridge, Mass.: Ballinger, 1974.

Malan, D. H. The most important development in psychotherapy since the discovery of the unconscious. In H. Davanloo (Ed.), *Short-term dynamic psychotherapy.* New York: Jason Aronson, 1980, pp. 13–24.

Mann, J. *Time limited psychotherapy.* Cambridge, Mass.: Harvard University Press, 1973.

Marmor, J. Short term dynamic psychotherapy. *American Journal of Psychiatry,* 1979, *136*(2), 149–155.

Martin, G. A., & Worthington, E. L. Behavioral homework. In M. Hersen, R. M. Eisler, & P. M. Miller (Eds.), *Progress in behavior modification* (Vol. 13). New York: Academic Press, in press.

Masters, W. H., & Johnson, V. E. *Human sexual inadequacy,* Boston: Little, Brown, 1980.

Minuchin, S. *Families and family therapy.* Cambridge, Mass.: Harvard University Press, 1974. (a)

Minuchin, S. Structural family therapy. In S. Arieti (Ed.), *American handbook of psychiatry* (Vol. III). New York: Basic Books, 1974, pp. 178–192. (b)

Minuchin, S., & Fishman, H. C. *Family therapy techniques.* Cambridge, Mass.: Harvard University Press, 1981.

Montalvo, B. (Therapist). In J. Haley & S. Scott (Eds.), *The family with a little fire.* Philadelphia: Philadelphia Child Guidance Clinic, 1973. (Videotape)

Munjack, D. J., & Oziel, R. J. Resistance in the behavioral treatment of sexual dysfunction. *Journal of Sex and Marital Therapy,* 1978, *4,* 122–138.

Papp, P. Paradoxical strategies and countertransference. In A. S. Gurman (Ed.), *Questions and answers in the practice of family therapy.* New York: Brunner/Mazel, 1981, pp. 201–203.

Papp. P. The Greek chorus and other techniques of paradoxical therapy. *Family Process,* 1980, *19*(1), 45–57.

Paul, N. L., & Grosser, G. Operational mourning and its role in conjoint family therapy. *Community Mental Health Journal,* 1965, *1*(4), 339–345.

Paul, N. L., & Paul, B. B. *A marital puzzle*. New York: W. W. Norton, 1975.

Rank, O. *Will therapy*. New York: Alfred A. Knopf, 1947.

Reiss, D., & Oliveri, M. D. Family paradigm and family coping: A proposal for linking the family's intrinsic adaptive capacities to its responses to stress. *Family Relations,* 1980, *29,* 431–444.

Reiss, D., & Sheriff, W. H. A computer-automated procedure for testing some experiences of family membership. *Behavioral Science,* 1970, *15*(5), 431–443.

Sager, C. J., Master, Y. J., Ronall, R. E., & Normand, W. C. Selection and engagement of patients in family therapy. *American Journal of Orthopsychiatry,* 1968, *38,* 715–723.

Selvini Palazzoli, M. Interview (translated from the German Newsletter *Kontext, 1,* 2). *The Underground Railroad,* 1981, *1,* 3.

Selvini Palazzoli, M., Boscolo, L., Cecchin, G., & Prata, G. *Paradox and counterparadox.* New York: Jason Aronson, 1978.

Selvini Palazzoli, M., Boscolo, L., Cecchin, G., & Prata, G. Hypothesizing–circularity–neutrality: Three guidelines for the conductor of the session. *Family Process,* 1980, *19*(1), 3–12.

Shapiro, R. J., & Budman, S. H. Defection, termination, and continuation in family and individual therapy. *Family Process,* 1973, *12,* 55–67.

Shelton, J. L., & Ackerman, J. M. *Homework in counseling and psychotherapy.* Springfield, Ill: Charles C Thomas, 1974.

Sifneos, P. E. *Short term psychotherapy and emotional crisis.* Cambridge, Mass.: Harvard University Press, 1973.

Skynner, A. C. R. An open-systems, group-analytic approach to family therapy. In A. S. Gurman & D. P. Kniskern (Eds.), *Handbook of family therapy.* New York: Brunner/ Mazel, 1981, pp. 39–84.

Solomon, M. A. A developmental, conceptual premise for family therapy. *Family Process,* 1973, *12,* 179–188.

Solomon, M. A. Resistance in family therapy: Some conceptual and technical considerations. *The Family Coordinator,* 1974, *23*(2), 159–163.

Speer, A. Family systems: Morphostasis and morphogenesis. *Family Process,* 1970, *9,* 259–278.

Spinks, S. H., & Birchter, G. Behavioral systems marital therapy: Dealing with resistance. *Family Process,* 1982, *21*(2), 169–186.

Stanton, M. D., Steier, F., & Todd, T. C. Paying families for attending sessions: Counteracting the dropout problem. *Journal of Marital and Family Therapy,* 1982, *8*(3), 371–373.

Stanton, M. D., & Todd, T. C. Engaging "resistant" families in treatment. *Family Process,* 1981, *20*(3), 261–293.

Starr, S. Dealing with common resistances to attending the first family therapy session. In A. S. Gurman (Ed.), *Questions and answers in the practice of family therapy.* New York: Brunner/Mazel, 1981, pp. 10–15.

Stierlin, H. *Psychoanalysis and family therapy.* New York: Jason Aronson, 1977.

Tennen, H., Rohrbaugh, M., Press, S., & White, L. Reactance theory and therapeutic paradox: A compliance–defiance model. *Psychotherapy: Theory, Research and Practice,* 1981, *18*(1), 14–22.

Tomm, K. Circularity: A preferred orientation for family assessment. In A. S. Gurman (Ed.), *Questions and answers in the practice of family therapy.* New York: Brunner/Mazel, 1981, pp. 84–87.

Van Deusen, J. M., Stanton, M. D., Scott, S. M., & Todd, T. C. Engaging resistant families in treatment: I. Getting the drug addict to recruit his family members. *International Journal of Addiction,* 1980, *15,* 1069–1089.

Walsh, F. (Ed.). *Normal family processes.* New York: Guilford Press, 1982.

Walsh, F. Famiiy therapy: A systemic orientation to treatment. In A. Rosenblatt & D. Wald-
fogel (Eds.), *Handbook of clinical social work*. San Francisco: Jossey-Bass, in press.
Whitaker, C. A., & Keith, D. V. Symbolic–experiential family therapy. In A. S. Gurman &
D. P. Kniskern (Eds.), *Handbook of family therapy*. New York: Brunner/Mazel,
1981, pp. 187–225.
Wilson, G. T., & Evans, I. M. The therapist–client relationship in behavior therapy. In A. S.
Gurman & A. M. Razin (Eds.), *Effective psychotherapy: A handbook of research.*
New York: Pergamon Press, 1977, pp. 283–301.
Wynne, L. C. The study of intrafamilial alignments and splits in exploratory family therapy.
In N. W. Ackerman, F. Beatman, & S. Sherman (Eds.), *Exploring the base for family
therapy*. New York: Family Service Association of America, 1961, pp. 95–115.
Wynne, L. C. Paradoxical interventions: Leverage for therapeutic change in individual and
family systems. In J. S. Strauss, M. Bowen, T. W. Downey, S. Fleck, S. Jackson, &
I. Levine (Eds.), *The psychotherapy of schizophrenia*. New York: Plenum Medical
Book Co., 1980, pp. 191–202.
Wynne, L. C., Ryckoff, I. M., Day, J., & Hirsch, S. I. Pseudo-mutuality in family relations
of schizophrenics. *Psychiatry, 1958, 21,* 205–220.

Index

Ackerman, J. M., 8, 9, 250*n*.
Ackerman, N. W., 14, 15, 247*n*.
Ackerman Institute, 21
Acting out, 130
  relabeling of, 198
Adminstrative aspects of therapy, 221,
    222, 235-238, 245
Adolescents, 44 (*see also* Children)
  dependency of, 28, 29
  silence and hostility of, 71, 72, 155, 174–
    178
  and therapist competence, 139, 140, 144
Age of therapists, 131, 132, 139, 140
Alexander, J., 19
Alliances
  nontherapeutic, 121-123
  therapeutic, 11, 34, 142, 215, 238
    and first interview, 56
    and responsibility for treatment, 37
American Association for Marriage and
    Family Therapists, 130
American Family Therapy Association,
    130
Analogies, use of in treatment, 233, 234
Anorexia nervosa, 3, 30, 51, 52, 98, 164
Antidepressant medication, 115
Anxiety, 5, 8, 10, 26, 27, 53, 64, 90, 96,
    115, 187, 221
  acknowledgment of, 97, 98
  and change, 147
  competence, 210-212, 227-229, 245
  and denial, 182, 183
  about deviancy, 92
  and ego strength, 7
  and hostility in therapy, 41, 176, 177
  and interruptions in first interview, 69
  minimization of in therapy, 16
  and motivation for therapy, 65, 104
  preparation for, 110
  in public speaking, 228, 229
  and receipt and processing of informa-
    tion, 30, 31
  and single-member dominance, 165-169

and symptoms, 234
and talkativeness, 165-169
of therapist, 104, 121, 146
  in first interview, 55
Aponte, H. J., 17, 18, 247*n*.
Ard, B., 14, 247*n*.
Arkowitz, H., 9, 249*n*.
Assertiveness training, 9
Attitudes of therapists, 219-221
Authority in therapy, 149, 180, 181
Avoidance, 13 (*see also* Denial)

Barker, P., 14*n*., 18, 247*n*.
Bateson, G., 20, 247*n*.
Beck, A., 11, 247*n*.
Behavioral treatment, 19, 20, 154, 231 (*see*
    also Reinforcement)
  and change, 8
  contracts in, 78
  of disruptive children, 172, 173
  strategies in, 8-10
Behavior modification (*see* Behavioral
    treatment)
Binge eating, 97
Bishop, D.S., 78, 247*n*.
Black-box approach, 13, 21
Borderline conditions, 90
Boscolo, L., 21, 250*n*.
Boszormenyi-Nagy, I., 13, 15, 16, 27, 178,
    247*n*.
Boundaries, family, 18, 119, 124, 213
  and contracts, 81
  early establishment of, 244, 245
  generational, 157, 163, 233
  negotiation of in first interview, 55-62
  rigidity of and denial, 183
  and roles and responsibilities, 219
Bowen, M., 15-17, 93, 178, 231, 247*n*.
Bradshaw, T., 64
Brehm, J. W., 31, 247*n*.
Burke, J. D., 7, 247*n*.
Burn out, professional, 214 (*see also* Fa-
    tigue of therapist)

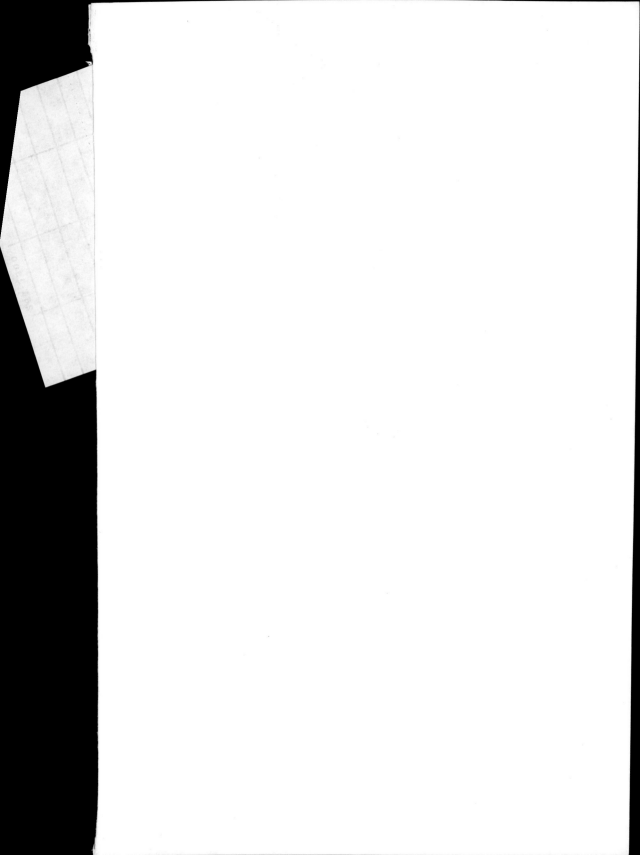